VITAMIN C

DEDICATION

To all students of nutrition: may you enjoy the subject and all its ramifications as much as we have. *Salute e buon appetito!*

VITAMIN C

The Mysterious Redox-System
A Trigger of Life?

Silvia Nobile, PhD, ARACI

and

Joan Mary Woodhill, RD, ScD

MTP PRESS LIMITED · LANCASTER · BOSTON · THE HAGUE
International Medical Publishers

Published in the UK and Europe by
MTP Press Limited
Falcon House
Lancaster, England

British Library Cataloguing in Publication Data

Nobile, S.
Vitamin C.
1. Vitamin C
I. Title II. Woodhill, J. M.
612'.399 QP772.A8

ISBN 978-94-011-9841-7 ISBN 978-94-011-9839-4 (eBook)
DOI 10.1007/978-94-011-9839-4

Published in the USA by
MTP Press
A division of Kluwer Boston Inc
190 Old Derby Street
Hingham, MA 02043, USA

Library of Congress Cataloging in Publication Data

Nobile, Sylvia, 1916–
Vitamin C: the mysterious redox-system – a trigger of life?

Includes bibliographical references and index.
1. Vitamin C. I. Woodhill, Joan Mary.
II. Title. (DNLM: 1. Ascorbic acid—Pharmacodynamics. QU 210 N745V)
QP772.A8N6 612'.399 81–14286
AACR2

Softcover reprint of the hardcover 1st edition 1981

Photoset, printed and bound in Great Britain by
REDWOOD BURN LIMITED
Trowbridge, Wiltshire

Contents

Preface 9

1 **Interactions, interdependence and interrelationships of vitamin C in human nutrition and metabolism** 11

2 **How was vitamin C discovered?** 15
- 2.1 Scurvy – historical background 15
- 2.2 Isolation of the antiscorbutic factor 16
- 2.3 Chemical and structural formulae and synthesis of vitamin C 16
- 2.4 Why cannot the human organism make its own vitamin C? 17
- 2.5 Naming names – vitamin C versus ascorbic acid 18

3 **What is vitamin C?** 21
- 3.1 Structure and physicochemical properties 21
- 3.2 Biochemical reactivity of the vitamin C system 24

4 **How is vitamin C determined?** 27
- 4.1 Assay of vitamin C in foods 27
- 4.2 Assay of vitamin C in human tissues and body fluids 29

5 **Where is vitamin C found? – vitamin C in foods** 31
- 5.1 Vitamin C in fruit and vegetables 32
- 5.2 Vitamin C in foods of animal origin 35

5.3 Standardization, restoration, enrichment or fortification of foods with L-ascorbic acid 36
5.4 Use of L-ascorbic acid as an antioxidant in foods 38
5.5 Assessment of food intake for vitamin C 38
5.6 Why food in preference to ascorbic acid tablets or crystalline ascorbic acid? 55

6 Vitamin C in the human body 57
6.1 Where does it go? 57
6.2 How does vitamin C function? 64
6.3 What does vitamin C do? 68

7 Case studies of scurvy and hypovitaminosis C in Australia 77
7.1 Mental performance of old men in a geriatric hospital 77
7.2 Mental performance of old men receiving meals-on-wheels 78
7.3 Precipitation of scurvy in an old woman 79
7.4 Aboriginal families and scurvy baby 80
7.5 Aboriginal women of childbearing age 80
7.6 Australian children from socioeconomic stress groups 81
7.7 Adult Australians in varying degrees of health 82

8 How much vitamin C do we humans need? – dietary allowances 87
8.1 Scurvy prevention versus tissue saturation – the great debate 88
8.2 Dietary allowances for vitamin C based on scurvy prevention 90
8.3 Dietary allowances for vitamin C based on the concept of approaching tissue saturation 93
8.4 The yo-yo of dietary allowances for vitamin C 94

9 Assessment of vitamin C status 97
9.1 Clinical, dietary and biochemical assessment 97
9.2 Correlations between clinical, dietary and biochemical vitamin C status in adults 100
9.3 Sex and age difference – intake and plasma levels of vitamin C 101

10 Vitamin C, modern lifestyle and hazards 105
10.1 Vitamin C in smoking and heavy drinking 105
10.2 Vitamin C and drugs 106
10.3 Vitamin C and climate 107

11 Dietary recommendations for the healthy man and woman of the 1980s 109

12 Ascorbic acid as a therapeutic agent – some controversial issues 111
12.1 Ascorbic acid and the common cold 112
12.2 Ascorbic acid and cancer 124
12.3 Ascorbic acid and atherosclerosis 125
12.4 Ascorbic acid and other diseases 125
12.5 Ascorbic acid and surgical trauma 125
12.6 Megadoses of ascorbic acid 125

13 Vitamin C and future research 133

14 Appendices 137
14.1 Summary of the fluorimetric determination of vitamin C in blood plasma 137
14.2 Examples of daily menus providing adequate vitamin C 139

15 References 145
15.1 Special references to vitamin C and the common cold 155

16 Abbreviations, Symbols and Glossary 161
16.1 Abbreviations 161
16.2 Symbols 162
16.3 Glossary 163

Index 179

Preface

Parents and ancestors are always important: they endow us with a genetic inheritance for better or for worse, for the balanced diet, for overfeeding or for starvation. Some of us die young, some succumb in middle age to chronic disease, others join the gerocracy – the healthy, happy people in their 70s, 80s or even 90s. Genetic inheritance, nurture and nutrition, all play their part. The nurture and nutrition are our own responsibility; we make our choices and live with the consequences.

This book is dedicated to the students of nutrition who may be interested in the subject for themselves alone, for their families, for teaching and counselling others and for research and investigations. We found it necessary to include basic information in order to support some of the statements we make or advice we give; this material appears either in the main body of the text or as footnotes. If the student of nutrition is familiar with the basic concepts, these sections can be skipped. At the end of the book we have included appendices, with examples of daily menus providing adequate vitamin C, an extensive bibliography, a glossary and an index. We have drawn up a food table of the vitamin C content of specific foods and described the point-system which is a ready-reckoner for approximate calculation of the vitamin C content of foods and diets. The book contains guidelines for the assessment of vitamin C status using dietary, biochemical and clinical yardsticks. Case studies on scurvy and hypovitaminosis C are reported.

The topic of vitamin C, as with many other scientific subjects, is controversial:

(1) The terminology itself is controversial; not all people accept that vitamin C is a redox-system containing at least three substances (L-ascorbic acid, monodehydro-L-ascorbic acid and dehydro-L-ascorbic acid) not just ascorbic acid.
(2) The amount of vitamin C needed by human beings to maintain optimum health and resistance to disease is disputed.
(3) Vitamin C and the common cold is a 'hot' topic.
(4) The use of megadoses of ascorbic acid is a 'burning' issue.

These are examples of particularly lively controversies about vitamin C, and hopefully the material in this book may help to clarify them. However, we feel that it is more important to throw further and brighter light on the mysterious functions of vitamin C in the human body rather than spend precious time and energy in producing sparks by raking over old coals.

1
Interactions, interdependence and interrelationships of vitamin C in human nutrition and metabolism

Nutrition can be regarded as the most ubiquitous environmental factor affecting human health and wellbeing and vitamin C is one of the most ubiquitous key nutrients.

Humans cannot produce vitamin C in their own bodies and must obtain it from food sources. 'Eat a mixed diet with a variety of foods' has been a slogan of nutrition education. Another slogan is: 'it is better to take vitamins in food rather than in pills', and this applies to vitamins in general and to vitamin C in particular because vitamin C interacts with, is interdependent upon, and is interrelated to several other nutrients. The mixed and varied diet must also be balanced; this means not only the right amount of the essential nutrients in relation to energy needs, but also the proper balance in relation to the functions in the body. Not too little, not too much – the right amount; too little or too much of one vitamin, day in and day out, could upset the balance of metabolic and enzyme functions.

The most outstanding properties of vitamin C are its solubility in water and its presence in plant and animal tissues as a redox-system (Figures 1 and 2). A redox-system is an oxidation–reduction system. Thus a substance such as ascorbic acid has the ability to give up hydrogen and become oxidized or to accept hydrogen and become reduced. Ascorbic acid is oxidized to dehydroascorbic acid which is also biologically active and the reaction is reversible. If oxidation continues beyond the dehydroascorbic

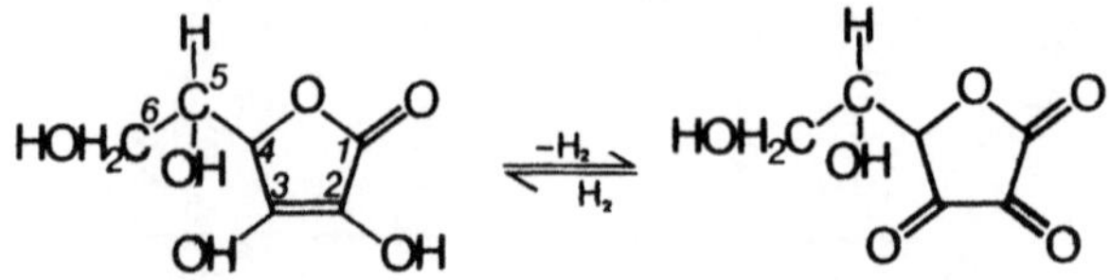

L-Ascorbic acid (reduced)

Dehydro-L-ascorbic acid (oxidized)

Figure 1 Vitamin C redox-system. Structural formulae of L-asorbic acid and dehydro-L-ascorbic acid

acid stage, the vitamin activity is lost. The vitamin C system is very unstable and the conditions of handling foods which contain this system, sensitive as it is to further oxidation, set the ground rules for retaining maximum vitamin C content throughout the whole food-handling chain.

The giving away and taking up of hydrogen by vitamin C is a most important metabolic function. There are many reactions of conversion from one substance to another in the vital processes of body metabolism that involve oxidation and reduction. Some of the relationships between vitamin C and other nutrients and metabolites are known but many others still have to be researched. Vitamin C plays an important part in the essential and sensitive balance in the workings of the body. It participates in the:

(1) hydrolysis of certain amino acids and is thus related to protein metabolism,
(2) formation of collagen or the intercellular cement substance necessary for body growth, tissue repair and wound healing,
(3) synthesis of the hormone adrenaline (epinephrine) and the hydroxylation of anti-inflammatory steroids in the adrenal gland,
(4) iron and copper metabolism, and
(5) folic acid metabolism (Marks, 1975).

The interactions of vitamin C with other vitamins has been studied extensively by Terroine (1960; 1966) with respect to animals. The investigations done so far on humans indicate that vitamin C is interrelated to the metabolism of the vitamins A, E, B_1 and B_{12} (Terroine, 1960, 1966).

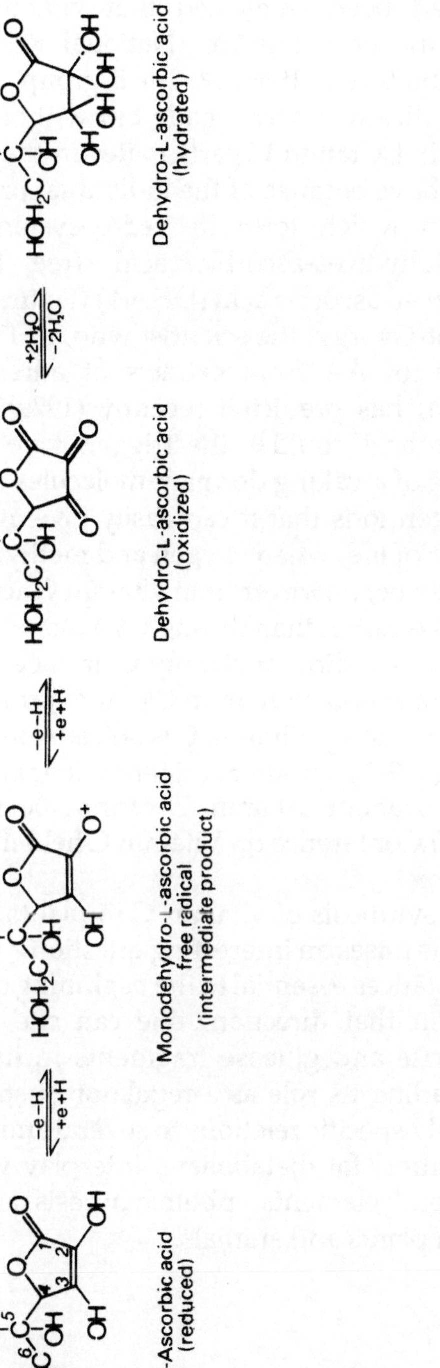

Figure 2 Vitamin C redox-system. Structural formulae of L-ascorbic acid, dehydro-L-ascorbic acid and the intermediate product monodehydro-L-ascorbic acid free radical

It had been suggested that vitamin C may function as a coenzyme or a cofactor (National Research Council Food and Nutrition Board, 1968) like the B-group vitamins and many studies in this direction were made but without success. It seems more likely that vitamin C participates in the metabolic pathways outlined above because of the individual properties of the three components which form its redox-system: L-ascorbic acid (AA), monodehydro-L-ascorbic acid free radical (MDHAA) and dehydro-L-ascorbic acid (DHAA) (Figure 2).

Szent-György, the scientist who, in 1928, obtained the first few crystals of AA from extracts of adrenal glands, cabbage and paprika, has predicted recently (1979) that vitamin C, through ascorbic acid, could be the 'trigger of life'. He postulated that AA is capable of awaking dormant molecules of protein by means of the hydrogen ions that it can easily give away, and thus ignites the process of life, when oxygen and methylglyoxal are present.

It may be, however, that vitamin C acts through the free radical MDHAA rather than through AA alone and, because the existence of this free radical of vitamin C has been ignored, the exact mechanism of action of vitamin C in the human body has eluded scientists for so long. Vitamin C is still surrounded by mystery.

King (1975), another eminent scientist whose early and later discoveries about vitamin C cannot be forgotten, in closing the Second Conference on Vitamin C held in 1974 in New York, said:

> The synthesis of vitamin C in plants, animals, and microorganisms raises an interesting question – was the vitamin one of the substances essential to the beginning of life on our planet? Pointing in that direction, one can cite the close relationship to glucose and glucose fragments in its origin and metabolism, including its role as a regulator of starch hydrolysis in plants, highly specific relations to several amino acids, proteins, several vitamins, fat metabolism, interplay with most of the essential mineral elements, photosynthesis and cellular respiration in both plants and animals.

2
How was vitamin C discovered?

2.1 SCURVY – HISTORICAL BACKGROUND

The disease scurvy has been known since antiquity and was prevalent in Northern Europe in the Middle Ages. It was a major cause of death of the crusaders, the explorers and the sailors on long voyages. There was no known cure for scurvy. Early observations were reported in the 16th century about the scurvy-preventive action of pine needles and the curative effects of lemon juice. Two centuries later Lind described in detail the symptoms of the disease and its prevention and cure by the inclusion of fresh fruit and vegetables in the diet. He also demonstrated that oranges and lemons were more effective than cider. Captain Cook made use of this information in his voyages and in the 18th and 19th centuries the Dutch and the English navy adopted the same scurvy-preventive measures (Rosenberg, 1945; Sherman, 1946). In the first decades of the 20th century the existence of food factors, essential for the treatment of certain diseases, was at last widely accepted. Factor A, found in butter and liver, was effective for the prevention and cure of xerophthalmia. Factor B, obtained from rice polishing, was a cure for beri-beri. The name 'vitamine' was proposed by Funk in 1912, who found that Factor B was an amine, and erroneously believed that all other accessory food factors essential for life (*vita*) were amines. Drummond in 1920 coined the word 'vitamin' and named factors A and B, vitamin A and vitamin

B respectively. Following the alphabet he called the antiscorbutic factor from oranges and lemons, vitamin C (Rosenberg, 1945).

2.2 ISOLATION OF THE ANTISCORBUTIC FACTOR

Budd in 1841 had predicted that the antiscorbutic activity of some foods was due to a definite substance. Many years elapsed before this could be demonstrated. A water-soluble, strongly reducing, optically active, white, crystalline compound was isolated by Szent-György in 1928 from cabbage, paprika and the adrenal glands of animals. He called this substance hexuronic acid. In the same year it was found to be identical with the antiscorbutic factor that had been isolated from lemon juice by Zilva (1923) and Waugh and King (1932). The substance was called first cevitamic acid then ascorbic acid. The existence of an equally active but oxidized compound was proven in that period (Zilva, 1927; Tillmans, 1930). It was called dehydroascorbic acid, and it was established that the two substances are interconvertible and form a redox-system.

2.3 CHEMICAL AND STRUCTURAL FORMULAE AND SYNTHESIS OF VITAMIN C

Szent-György had determined the empirical formula of hexuronic acid (ascorbic acid) as $C_6H_8O_6$ and with Haworth in 1933 established its structure as a monosaccharide sugar – the 2, 3 dienol-L-gulonic acid lactone. In modern chemical language this is called the L-threo-2,3,4,5,6 pentahydroxy-1-hexenoic acid-4-lactone (Figure 1). L-Ascorbic acid forms a redox-system with its first oxidation product the dehydro-L-ascorbic acid, the chemical formula of which is $C_6H_6O_6$ (Figure 1). The existence of an intermediate product of the oxidation reaction, the monodehydro-L-ascorbic acid free radical was postulated in 1938 by Bezssonoff and Woloszyn and established in later studies (Yamazaki, Mason, and Piette, 1959, 1960; Yamazaki and Piette, 1961). It has the chemical formula $C_6H_7O_6$ (Figure 2).

Knowledge of the chemical structure allowed the production of L-ascorbic acid by synthesis. The starting material for the synthesis was either glucose, galactose, other simple sugars or a ketosugar like L-sorbose (Reichstein and Grüssner, 1934). It was the first vitamin to be synthesized industrially and thus made available in large amounts for use in therapy and research studies. Dehydro-L-ascorbic acid may be obtained in the laboratory by controlled oxidation of L-ascorbic acid, for example, with iodine. Monodehydro-L-ascorbic acid is a free radical, that is, a very transient compound, which is formed from either L-ascorbic acid or dehydro-L-ascorbic acid in high energy ionizing radiation and enzymatic and non-enzymatic redox-reactions (Bielski, Richter, and Chan, 1975; Lewin, 1976; Sebrell and Harris, 1967).

2.4 WHY CANNOT THE HUMAN ORGANISM MAKE ITS OWN VITAMIN C?

The human organism cannot make its own vitamin C because through evolution and genetic mutation it has lost a particular enzyme system (L-gulono-γ-lactone oxidase) which can transform a sugar like glucose or galactose into ascorbic acid. Thus all human beings must rely upon outside sources of vitamin C to cover their needs. However, they are not the only animal species with this problem. A group of Indian scientists (Chatterjee *et al.*, 1961; 1975) found that insects, invertebrates and fishes which are at the bottom end of the evolutionary tree, and guinea pigs, the flying mammals (bats) and monkeys which follow man from the top end of the evolutionary tree have also lost the particular enzyme system and thus cannot make their own vitamin C. All other animals* so far studied possess the enzyme system and can produce vitamin C when needed. For them too evolution has played a part because lower animals like amphibians (toads, frogs) and reptiles (turtles, lizards, snakes, tortoises) have the particular enzyme system in the kidneys. In the mammals, however (for example, goats, cows, sheep, rats, mice, rabbits, cats and dogs) the enzyme system has changed location from kidneys to liver. Birds are said to have evolved from reptiles and have a similar pattern to the mammals as to the location or loss of the enzyme system. The primitive birds have it in the kidneys, like the reptiles; some birds (such as the house crow) share it between kidneys and liver. More evolved birds, the passeriform, have it only in the

*Nothing is known about Australian marsupials and other animals as to their capacity to make or not to make their own vitamin C. It has been observed that the Australian opossum attacks fruit and the parsley beds, and the flying foxes swarm into the loquat and prunus trees.

liver, and the top class of passeres (for example, the jungle bubbler) do not have it at all (see Figure 3).

It seems that man has lost the gene responsible for producing the enzyme system, and hence vitamin C, some 25 million years ago. Evolution has relieved man of the burden of synthesizing the vitamin in his own organism but has made him dependent on his environment for obtaining vitamin C. This vitamin is essential to man's growth and wellbeing and without it he would die of scurvy like the sailors on long voyages in the past.

2.5 NAMING NAMES – VITAMIN C VERSUS ASCORBIC ACID

The chemical name (see Section 2.3) was too long and meaningless for common use and thus the 'trivial' name ascorbic acid was accepted as an alternative name for vitamin C (a = anti, scorbic = an abbreviation of scorbutic, the adjective pertaining to scurvy). However L-ascorbic acid is not the only substance possessing vitamin C activity. Its first oxidation product, the dehydro-L-ascorbic acid and the intermediate product of the oxidation, the monodehydro-L-ascorbic acid free radical have an antiscorbutic activity equal to L-ascorbic acid.

In plant and animal tissues all three forms of L-ascorbic acid may be found and, since all forms are active, they must be considered when determining the vitamin C content of foods and animal tissues. For this reason there is no better term than *Vitamin* C for expressing the sum of biologically active ascorbic acid derivatives (Nobile, 1974a). When reference is made to the individual components it is appropriate to give them the 'trivial' names: L-ascorbic acid – or in short, AA; dehydro-L-ascorbic acid – or in short, DHAA; and monodehydro-L-ascorbic acid free radical – or in short, MDHAA. Some people think it sounds scientific and scholarly to call vitamin C ascorbic acid. Its discoverers adopted this as a 'trivial' name (in other words, the vernacular name or made-up name) to describe the antiscorbutic vitamin. To use the term ascorbic acid for vitamin C is not correct. Those people who persist in trying to sound scientific by using the term ascorbic acid when they mean vitamin C show that they do not understand the basic and most important biochemical function of vitamin C, that is donating and receiving hydrogen ions to and from many

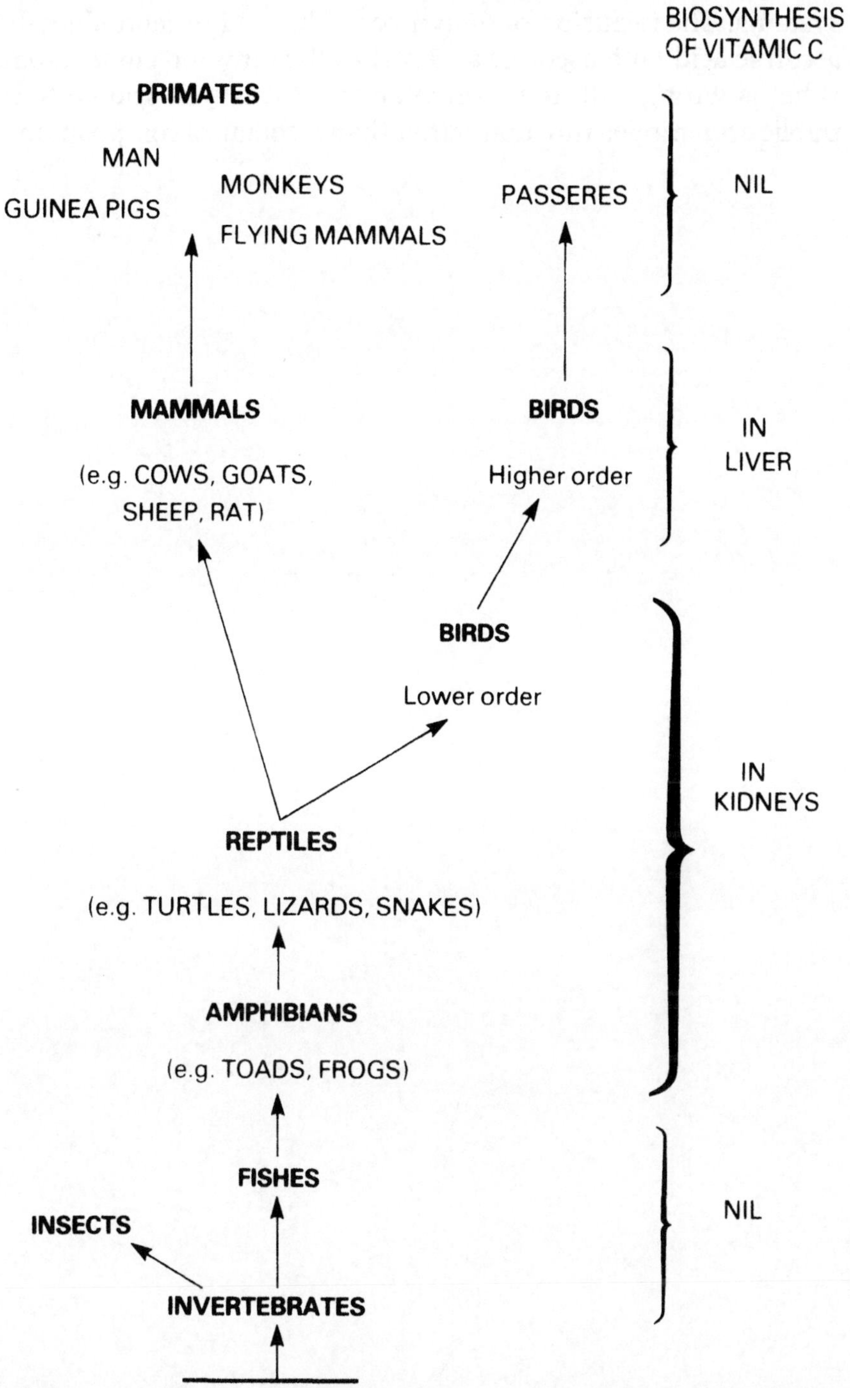

Figure 3 Vitamin C biosynthesis in the evolutionary process (adapted from Chatterjee *et al.*, 1961, 1975)

systems. The inclusion of dehydroascorbic and/or monodehydroascorbic acid with ascorbic acid makes the term too cumbersome. What is wrong with the term vitamin C? It is well known to the public and implies function rather than a chemical composition.

3
What is vitamin C?

3.1 STRUCTURE AND PHYSICOCHEMICAL PROPERTIES

Vitamin C is a redox-system comprising L-ascorbic acid (AA), the free radical monodehydro-L-ascorbic acid (MDHAA) and dehydro-L-ascorbic acid (DHAA) (Figure 2). The three substances are interconvertible but each has distinct individual physicochemical properties (Sebrell and Harris, 1967; Lewin, 1976), some of which have been summarized in Table 1.

The structure of the vitamin C system is essentially planar. Each of the three components has, in its molecule, a lactone ring* one keto-group (C=O) in C-1, and two hydroxyl-groups (OH) in C-5 and C-6. The carbon atom in C-5 is asymmetric; the space orientation of its H and OH groups and the ring structure of the molecule are responsible for the *positive optical rotation* of AA and DHAA. The optical rotation of MDHAA is not known. The optical rotation of AA increases upon addition of alkali (for example, sodium hydroxide) to its water solution which results in the formation of salts (for example, sodium ascorbate). The presence of a double bond in the ring confers upon AA and MDHAA their *absorption properties* in the ultraviolet (UV) light region. The absorption spectrum of AA has one maximum at 244–245 nm which moves to 265 nm in the presence of alkali. MDHAA shows a main maximum at 360 nm and another maximum at 285–310 nm which

*C-1 and C-4 are linked with an atom of oxygen.

Table 1 Physicochemical properties of vitamin C

Substance	*Optical rotation* $[\alpha]_D^{20°}$	*UV spectrum* λ max. nm	ε max.	*Melting point* °C	*Redox-system*	*Redox potential (volts) at pH 7.0*
L-Ascorbic acid (AA)	+ 23°	244(pH 1.5)	10 500	192 decomp.	DHAA → AA	+ 0.058
Dehydro-L-ascorbic acid (DHAA)	+ 55°	300 ?	720	225 decomp.	AA → DHAA	− 0.058
Monodehydro-L-ascorbic acid free radical (MDHAA)	?	360 (pH 9.0)	?	?	MDHAA → AA	+ 0.34
Sodium ascorbate	+ 106°	265 (pH 7.4)	20 400	220 decomp.	MDHAA → DHAA	?

moves to higher wavelengths with increasing acidity of the solution (Bielski, Richter and Chan, 1975). DHAA has no double bond system in the ring and shows only a very weak absorption at 300 nm. AA is readily soluble in water (approximately 30 g of AA dissolve in 100 ml of water) from which it crystallizes as square or oblong crystals which *melt* at 192 °C with decomposition. The crystals are stable at room temperature and in the absence of air and moisture. DHAA melts at about 225 °C and is less soluble in water but more soluble than AA in lower alcohols, such as butanol. The crystals of DHAA are unstable to air. Solubility and melting point of MDHAA are not known. The two hydroxyl-groups (OH) in position C-2 and C-3 of the AA molecule are different from the other OH-groups at C-5 and C-6 with respect to their acidic properties. An 0.5% solution of AA in water is strongly acidic with a pH of 3.0, but DHAA in the oxidized form does not act as an acid because it does not have the two OH-groups in C-2 and C-3. *Ionization* of AA in water solutions occurs in two stages at the C-2 and C-3 OH-groups, and depends upon the pH of the solution. The first dissociation constant – pK – value is 4.18 and the second pK value is 11.6 at 37 °C and similar values were reported at 16 °C and 18 °C. Ionization of DHAA occurs with a pK value of approximately 9.0. This indicates that DHAA exists also in a hydrated form, for example, with two OH-groups each at C-2 and C-3 as indicated in Figure 2 (Lewin, 1976). The *stability* of AA in pure water solutions is greater at pH below 4.0 than in the alkaline pH range. DHAA is less stable than AA at any pH and MDHAA, which may be found over the entire pH range (0–13), appears more stable at pH 8.0 to 10.0 (Bielski, Richter and Chan, 1975). *Irradiation* of alkaline solutions of AA with either X-rays, gamma-rays or UV-light produces MDHAA, DHAA and hydrogen peroxide under both aerobic and anaerobic conditions. The two OH-groups at C-1 and C-2 of the AA molecule are bound by a double bond and are capable of *donating and receiving hydrogen*. In water solution AA is rapidly *oxidized* by atmospheric oxygen and other oxidizing agents to DHAA. In the presence of compounds containing –SH-groups such as glutathione DHAA is easily *reduced* to AA. This reversible reaction forms the redox-system of vitamin C. The intermediate product of the oxidation reaction of AA to DHAA, the MDHAA free radical, has both reducing and oxidizing properties and can be either reduced to AA or oxidized to DHAA. The *redox potential* or standard oxidation-reduction potential of the redox-system of vitamin C (AA⇋ DHAA) is ± 0.058 volts at pH 7.0 (Ball, 1937). The redox potential of the reduction of MDHAA to AA is more positive (about +0.34 volts) than that of the reduction of DHAA to AA (+ 0.058 volts). The redox potential of the oxidation of MDHAA to DHAA is not known (Lewin, 1976). The redox-system of vitamin C is very unstable and in the presence of strong oxidizing agents oxidation may continue beyond the DHAA stage and destroy the biological activity of vitamin C with the formation of various inactive compounds. The rate of *oxidative destruction* of the vitamin C system is pH-dependent; it is more rapid in alkaline than in acid media, and is catalysed by even traces of copper and iron, and accelerated by heat and UV light. The *nature of the oxidation products* of ascorbic acid is also pH-dependent and varies with the alkali used. MDHAA, DHAA and hydrogen peroxide are formed on oxidation of AA by atmospheric oxygen which may be catalysed by UV light and the presence of even traces of copper. Inactive products such as oxalic acid are found during auto-oxidation of AA in alkaline solutions but not at pH 4.0 or below. Diketo-L-gulonic acid results from hydrolytic rupture of the lactone ring. L-Lyxonic acid, L-xylonic acid and L-threonic acid are some of the identified inactive compounds resulting from the destruction of the redox-system, but there are other such compounds still awaiting identification.

All the factors which affect the stability of vitamin C should be considered whenever maximum preservation of vitamin C in foods is required (see Chapter 5) and in the transport and storage of plant and animal tissues for analysis and during the analytical determination of the vitamin (see Chapter 4). Absence of air and metals, maintenance of low temperature and acid conditions, avoidance of contact with copper and iron which may be derived from food containers or cooking pots are the most essential precautions which food processors, cooks and analysts must always bear in mind when dealing with vitamin C.

3.2 BIOCHEMICAL REACTIVITY OF THE VITAMIN C SYSTEM

The individual physicochemical and redox properties of ascorbic acid (AA), monodehydroascorbic acid free radical (MDHAA), and dehydroascorbic acid (DHAA) outlined in Section 3.1 are of basic importance in the understanding of the biochemical reactions occurring within the human body and involving vitamin C.

AA is more soluble in water than DHAA and is the main component of vitamin C in the plasma and other body fluids. Contrary to the *in vitro* performance at neutral pH, AA in the plasma appears to be stable. It may be present as its sodium salt and is probably protected by the physiological concentration of sodium chloride in the plasma or it may be stabilized through binding with some proteins (Bogdanov and Zviagina, 1975; Lewin, 1976). In watery media AA is ionized and, as an anion it can form salts with cations such as sodium (Na), ammonium (NH_4) and calcium (Ca). In the routine treatment of spinally injured patients large doses of AA are prescribed to acidify the urine because the excess AA facilitates removal, by excretion, of the alkali present. AA may form complexes with metallic cations, such as iron (Fe), copper (Cu), magnesium (Mg), and in this way it may interact in the metabolism of these metals.

DHAA is the hydrophobic component of the vitamin C system as it has more lipid-like properties than AA and possesses a greater power to reduce interfacial tension. Thus vitamin C acts as a metabolic detergent and may dissolve fats, cholesterol and cholesterol–phospholipid–calcium complexes (Lewin, 1976). DHAA increases membrane permeability and penetrates lipoid membranes* more readily than AA and by its presence DHAA facilitates the permeability of the membranes to AA. DHAA is easily reduced to AA by compounds containing –SH-groups, such as glutathione, which are essential to the maintenance of the redox-system of vitamin C in equilibrium. In certain physiological malfunction, for example, infectious diseases, hyperthyroidism (Banerjee, 1977) and diabetes (Chatterjee *et al.*, 1975), low blood levels of glutathione and AA accompanied by abnormally high levels of DHAA are found. Banerjee (1977) reports similar findings after injection of thyroxin, corticotrophin and cortisone but states that no DHAA could be detected in the blood after continued administration of a large dose of AA. He indicates that DHAA may have a role in controlling cell division. Chatterjee *et al.* (1975) consider that the accumulation of DHAA in diabetic patients accompanied by high levels of blood

*For example, the membranes of the erythrocytes (red blood cells) and of the eye and brain cells.

sugar may be due to increased rate of oxidation of AA. The resulting DHAA may act with the –SH-amino acids which are essential for the biosynthesis of insulin thus inhibiting its formation.

The biochemical reactivity of the free radical *MDHAA* is its ability to act as an oxidizing or as a reducing agent in appropriate redox-systems involving vitamin C (Lewin, 1976). Lewin states that the thermodynamic equilibrium conditions, so far believed to be basic for evaluating the direction of oxidations or reductions, are applicable to simple biochemical systems but not to complex ones. The participation of the vitamin C redox-system in many complex biochemical reactions can be explained only by the intervention of excess MDHAA. High MDHAA concentrations are attained in certain enzymatic reactions involving vitamin C, and enzymes such as peroxidase and ascorbic acid oxidase (Yamazaki, Mason, and Piette, 1959). MDHAA possesses higher energy levels than AA as it has one unpaired electron (Figure 2). It is therefore often via MDHAA that vitamin C takes part in electron transfer, energy transfer, certain hydroxylation reactions (such as dopamine to noradrenaline), in the reduction of cytochrome-*c*, in the activation of NADH oxidase (nicotinamide-adenine dinucleotide reduced), in the deactivation of toxic substances (for example, adrenochromes in the adrenal glands), in the maintenance of active –SH-groups (which are low in physiological malfunctions) and in the protection of the cyclic nucleotides cAMP (cyclic adenosine 3′,5′-monophosphate) and cGMP (cyclic guanosine 3′,5′-monophosphate) (Lewin, 1976). These cyclic nucleotides are involved in various hormonal and physiological activities and in the synthesis of a number of enzymes.

4
How is vitamin C determined?

Before attempting a determination of vitamin C in any type of products it is important to realize and always remember that vitamin C is a redox-system and therefore very unstable. It is useless to determine vitamin C unless strict precautions are taken in the laboratory to protect the vitamin before and during the analytical procedure. It is recommended:

(1) to use bidistilled water for the preparation of the reagents in order to avoid contamination with any metal,
(2) to use metaphosphoric acid for extracting the vitamin because it is the best known stabilizer for vitamin C,
(3) to avoid using alkali, heat and exposing samples and extracts of the vitamin to UV light at any stage of the assay,
(4) to avoid contact with air as far as possible or the use of any oxidizing agent which may destroy the vitamin beyond the dehydroascorbic acid stage.

4.1 ASSAY OF VITAMIN C IN FOODS

Collection and preparation of samples for assay

Samples of foods which are collected outside the laboratory, such as in nutritional surveys, must be placed in opaque plastic containers tightly sealed and immediately deep frozen by means of dry ice (solid carbon dioxide) in an insulated container. The samples should be transported to the laboratory as soon as feasible, where they should be homogenized immediately and rapidly in the presence of a solution of metaphosphoric acid (usually 5%). This is achieved by weighing an aliquot of the food, and adding to it a quantity, by weight, of metaphosphoric acid solution suitable to produce, after homogenization, a free-flowing slurry, ready for assay. If assay cannot be performed immediately the homogenized samples, in appropriate and tightly sealed containers, should be stored in the deep freeze at −20 °C or lower, for no longer than 3 months. Thawing of the samples before assay should be done only once and at room temperature, or by placing the samples overnight in the refrigerator at +4 °C.

Biological assays

These tests, using vitamin C-deficient guinea-pigs as test animals, were developed in the early period of vitamin C research to determine the amount of the vitamin which was necessary to cure and/or prevent the onset of scurvy-deficiency symptoms. The tests most frequently used were based on the assessment of dental changes and growth of the deficient animals. These assays were expensive and time-consuming and were eventually replaced by physicochemical procedures which, however, do not measure the biological availability of the vitamin. The early Food Composition Tables published in Australia by CSIR (Council for Scientific and Industrial Research) (Marston and Dawbarn, 1941) report values for vitamin C in foods found by the dichlorophenol indophenol method and state that some of the values were confirmed by biological assays.

Physicochemical methods

Several physicochemical methods are available for determining vitamin C in foods but no method has yet been developed which would allow the simultaneous determination of ascorbic acid (AA) and dehydroascorbic acid (DHAA). The procedures based on the reaction of AA with oxidizing agents such as 2,6-dichlorophenol indophenol or iodine do not measure DHAA and therefore should not be used in the assay of vitamin C. Such tests are useful to assay tablets, solutions, or other products known to contain only AA. The most specific methods so far available for the assay of vitamin C (AA + DHAA) in foods are based on the controlled oxidation of AA to DHAA after extraction of the vitamin from the food with metaphosphoric acid to ensure its stability during assay. DHAA is then coupled with 2,4-dinitrophenylhydrazine to form a coloured derivative which is purified by column and thin layer chromatography before measurement (Vuillemier, 1967). Alternatively, the fluorimetric method of Deutsch and Weeks (1965) based on the reaction between *o*-phenylene diamine and DHAA and the formation of a fluorescent quinoxaline derivative, may be applied to foods. In laboratories where the instrument is available vitamin C could be determined by high pressure liquid chromatography (HPLC) after purification of the extract. This procedure has high detection limits and specificity (Williams, Baker, and Schmit, 1973; Floridi *et al.*, 1981).

4.2 ASSAY OF VITAMIN C IN HUMAN TISSUES AND BODY FLUIDS

Collection and preparation of samples for assay

Human tissues (for example, biopsy samples obtained from living patients or at post-mortem) should be homogenized with metaphosphoric acid immediately after sampling or else kept deep-frozen until preparation for assay can be performed as described in Section 4.1. Assay should be carried out as soon as possible because vitamin C in tissues is very unstable. Solid metaphosphoric acid should be added to samples of *urine* to achieve a final concentration of the acid of 5%. This treatment should be done as soon as the samples are obtained to avoid destruction of vitamin C through changes in pH. Then the mixture should be kept deep-frozen prior to assay. Venous *blood* from fasting subjects should be drawn directly into heparinized syringes (heparin prevents clotting) mixed gently and centrifuged immediately for 5 min. The *plasma* which separates on top of the blood cells (leukocytes, platelets and erythrocytes) should be clear, pale-coloured and have no trace of haemolysis. If assay of vitamin C is to be carried out in the plasma it should be treated immediately with a 5% solution of metaphosphoric acid (for instance, 1 ml plasma plus 9 ml acid), mixed thoroughly and stored deep-frozen. Before assay the mixture should be allowed to thaw only once, centrifuged and the vitamin C measured in the clear supernatant solution. Preparation of the *buffy coat* (white blood cells and platelets) of the *leukocytes*, of the *platelets* and the *red blood cells* for the assay of vitamin C is more elaborate and should not be attempted unless an exact count of the blood cells can be performed (for instance, using a Coulter counter). Description of such methods is reported by Gyorgy (1950). Loh and Wilson (1971a) described an improved method for testing vitamin C in leukocytes, Attwood *et al.* (1974) proposed a special technique to determine vitamin C in leukocytes and platelets which does not require separation of the cells, and Fazio, Wahlqvist, and Flint (1979) developed a new procedure for the preparation of platelets.

Measurement of vitamin C in human tissues and body fluids is best performed either by colorimetry using 2,4-dinitrophenylhydrazine or by fluorimetry with *o*-phenylene diamine after controlled oxidation of ascorbic acid (AA) to dehydroascorbic acid (DHAA) as outlined in Section 4.1. The fluorimetric method for determining vitamin C in blood plasma is summarized in Appendix 1.

High pressure liquid chromatography (HPLC) could also be applied. It is to be hoped that a HPLC technique will be developed to allow simultaneous and separate determination, in tissues and body fluids, of at least ascorbic acid and dehydroascorbic acid and possibly of other components of the vitamin C system. This information is needed to establish the ratio of AA to DHAA in each tissue or fluid. Recent work (Banerjee, 1977; Chatterjee *et al.*, 1975) showed that increased levels of DHAA in blood may be indicative of physiological malfunction. To obtain this information with present techniques it is necessary to measure, in the same sample, AA by the dye titration method and AA + DHAA as explained above and calculate DHAA by difference.

5
Where is vitamin C found? – vitamin C in foods

The main sources of vitamin C are fruit and vegetables but some foods of animal origin contain more than traces of the vitamin.

Whether or not we can obtain enough vitamin C from the modern diet depends upon how the food-handlers and the cooks treat the food on its way from the orchards and market gardens to the consumers' meal tables. Modern storage methods, processing and cooking practices can destroy vitamin C in the food.

Vitamin C is:

(1) an elusive vitamin: sometimes it is there in food, sometimes it is not;
(2) very variable in concentration even in the food groups (fruit and vegetables) that are recognized as good sources of the vitamin; some fruit and vegetables are good sources of vitamin C while others have only a negligible content, even when freshly harvested;
(3) very soluble in water and very sensitive to alkali;
(4) very sensitive to oxidation and heat;
(5) very sensitive to the presence of copper and iron; these elements hasten the destruction of vitamin C by catalysing oxidation reactions.

5.1 VITAMIN C IN FRUIT AND VEGETABLES

As vitamin C is a simple sugar, it is not surprising that it dissolves readily in water. It is found in fruit and vegetables, all of which have a high proportion of their weight as water. Vitamin C can easily diffuse out of this watery medium particularly if the cell walls are damaged. The contribution of any fruit and vegetable to the vitamin C content of the diet varies depending on the climate, the conditions of the soil, seasonal variations, the degree of maturity, the freshness of the food and the part of it which is eaten. The skin of apples, for instance, contains more vitamin C than the pulp. During *maturation* peas lose a considerable amount of vitamin C but this does not occur in tubers such as potatoes, nor in leafy vegetables such as spinach. During *storage* after harvesting, the vitamin C content of fruit and vegetables will decrease depending on the time and temperature conditions of storage and the type of food. Soft berries and green vegetables rapidly lose their vitamin C content due to bruising. Hard fruit and root vegetables can be stored without great losses of the vitamin. New potatoes are good sources of vitamin C but their content declines slowly during storage and may be reduced to about ⅙ of the original amount after 8 or 9 months (see Table 2).

Damaged tissues

The vitamin C content of sliced, cut or bruised fruit and vegetables diminishes rapidly when such foods are left standing or if washed with water. Cabbage, for instance, is an excellent source of vitamin C. But when cabbage is shredded, the cell walls are damaged and an enzyme which is normally present in the cells, called ascorbic acid oxidase, is released. It oxidizes the vitamin C beyond the dehydroascorbic acid stage and all that remains are the oxidized products of vitamin C which no longer possess vitamin C activity. The rate of enzymatic oxidation increases as the cooking temperature is raised but the enzyme is destroyed when the temperature reaches boiling point. Plunging the vegetable into boiling water or blanching it should preserve vitamin C by destroying ascorbic acid oxidase. Vitamin C is water-soluble and there are many cut cells in shredded cabbage; if shredded cabbage is left to soak for long periods, after scalding with boiling water, vitamin C will leach out and be thrown away with the water. Bruising vegetables will also

Table 2 Percentage losses of vitamin C during storage (a) and cooking (b) of potatoes and in the processing of peas (c)

(a) *Storage of raw potatoes* (Paul and Southgate, 1978)

Storage time	*Vitamin C* mg/100 g	*% Loss*
Potatoes raw freshly dug	30	0
Stored 1–3 months	20	33
Stored 4–5 months	15	50
Stored 6–7 months	10	67
Stored 8–9 months	8	73

(b) *Cooking of potatoes* (Paul and Southgate, 1978)

Method of cooking potatoes	*% Loss*
Boiled, peeled; Mashed	30–50
Boiled, unpeeled; Baked; Roasted; Steamed	20–40
Fried in deep fat (chips)	25–35

(c) *Processing of peas* (Mapson, 1956): vitamin C content of fresh raw peas (15–35 mg/100 g) (Paul and Southgate, 1978)

Fresh	*% Loss*	*Frozen*	*% Loss*	*Canned*	*% Loss*	*Air-dried*	*% Loss*	*Freeze-dried*	*% Loss*
		Scalding	25	Scalding	30	Scalding	25	Scalding	25
		Freezing	25	Heat sterilization	37	Drying	55	Drying	30
		Thawing	29	Diffusion into liquor	60				
Cooking	56	Cooking	61	Heating	64	Cooking	75	Cooking	65

activate ascorbic acid oxidase, so bruised tomatoes, for example, would contain less vitamin C than sound unblemished ones. Further and considerable losses of vitamin C will occur after boiling the sliced, cut or bruised vegetables and fruit especially when the boiling water is discarded and the cooked foods are then kept hot for a long time, as in large-scale catering.

Effects of pH of cooking media

In the early decades of this century, it was a common cooking practice to add bicarbonate of soda to peas and beans to retain the green colour (Elger, 1980). This softens the cell walls and makes the cooking water more alkaline. An alkaline pH would have a marked influence on the stability of vitamin C. So the more bicarbonate of soda added, the more vitamin C will be destroyed during cooking.

Jam and marmalade making

Boiling of fruit in the presence of sugar destroys only little vitamin C, provided the fruit is not damaged and is freshly processed after harvesting, and is not cooked in copper or iron pots.

Scalding, blanching, canning and bottling

Scalding and blanching is a process used to treat vegetables before canning, freezing or dehydration to remove undesirable gases and to inactivate enzymes, such as ascorbic acid oxidase, which would otherwise destroy vitamin C. The process consists of plunging the vegetables briefly into boiling water or exposing them to steam.

Canning and bottling of vegetables and fruit does not in itself cause noticeable losses of vitamin C. These may occur due to either oxidation or leaching out of the vitamin, but may be reduced if the foods are rapidly cooled (such as by cold air) immediately after scalding. Losses of vitamin C however increase if the fruit or vegetable is cut into small pieces.

Heat sterilization, freezing, irradiation and chemical preservatives

Heat sterilization of the sealed cans inactivates completely the enzymes which would destroy vitamin C. During storage, after canning, the remaining vitamin C content of the foods is sufficiently stable up to 1 to 2 years.

Freezing, after scalding, is a good method for preserving the vitamin C content of foods because the enzymes are almost completely inactivated and losses of vitamin C are kept to a minimum. However, very great losses of the vitamin occur on thawing and rethawing of frozen foods. Dehydration by freeze-drying protects vitamin C and only minor losses may occur in factory-dried vegetables such as peas (see Table 2). Irradiation has been used to sterilize food although at times it may cause undesirable changes in flavour and vitamin C is very sensitive to this method.

Chemical preservatives such as sulphites are often used to protect vitamin C from oxidation during pasteurization of juices or blanching of processed fruit, fruit juices, dried fruit and vegetables. Benzoates do not destroy vitamin C but do not protect it either, as they are not anti-oxidants and, in fruit juices, cannot prevent any dissolved oxygen from oxidizing vitamin C (Sebrell and Harris, 1967). Losses of vitamin C which have been reported to occur during various food processing methods are summarized in Table 2 taking peas as an example (Mapson, 1956).

In the assessment of the vitamin C content of the diet it is important to know the history of the food in order to evaluate the losses that may have occurred before the food is consumed. A comparison between the vitamin C content of vegetables, as eaten, cooked in institutions or in small households is illustrated in Figure 4, where the values found on analysis of vitamin C or calculated from Food Composition Tables are reported (Woodhill and Nobile, 1972/1973). Table 2 shows the losses of vitamin C which may occur in potatoes cooked by various methods (Paul and Southgate, 1978).

5.2 VITAMIN C IN FOODS OF ANIMAL ORIGIN

Vitamin C is found in tissues of high metabolic activity, both of animals which can make the vitamin in their own body and of those which must obtain it from outside sources. It is present in the eyes, the adrenals, other endocrine glands, the ovaries, spleen, lungs, liver, brain, kidneys, heart muscle, spinal fluid, blood and all blood cells, and milk. Breast milk contains normally about three

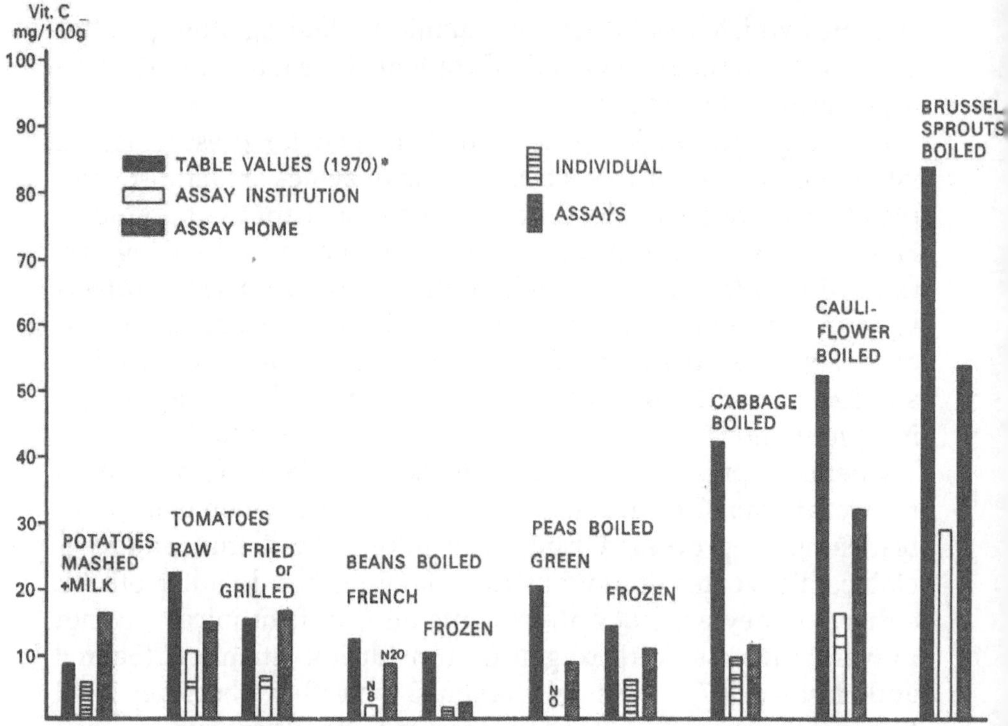

Figure 4 Vitamin C in institutional and home cooking (from Woodhill and Nobile, 1972/1973, with permission)

times the amount of vitamin C of cow's milk (Paul and Southgate, 1978). The consumption of liver, brain, kidneys and other offal may make a considerable contribution to the vitamin C content of a meal, provided these items are bought fresh and cooked with care (see Table 3, page 39). Losses of vitamin C occur during pasteurization, sterilization and dehydration of milk.

5.3 STANDARDIZATION, RESTORATION, ENRICHMENT OR FORTIFICATION OF FOODS WITH L-ASCORBIC ACID

Standardization

The Pure Food Act of New South Wales (1977) states that the following pure fruit juices should contain not less than the given amount of vitamin C, namely:

Juice	*Minimum concentration of vitamin* C (in mg/100 ml)
Orange	40
Lemon	35
Grapefruit	30
Orange and grapefruit	35
Blackcurrant	70
Pineapple	10

Any concentrate of these juices must contain, when diluted, at least the amount of vitamin C stated. As the vitamin C content of fresh fruit may vary widely and if pure juices do not contain the concentration required, L-ascorbic acid may be added to the juices to achieve the standard amount.

Restoration

This means adding to the food the amount of a nutrient which has been lost during any food processing (for example, milling of wheat which entails a reduction in several of the B vitamins originally present). In the case of vitamin C, restoration of the losses which may occur during storage, freezing, cooking, etc., of vegetables and fruit is not feasible unless food is preserved or bottled. A food in which the vitamin C content could be restored to the initial level is full cream and skim milk powder.

Enrichment or fortification

This is a term used when a nutrient is added to a food in an amount in excess of that naturally present. Some brand of instant potatoes may be fortified with L-ascorbic acid to contain about ten times the amount normally present – for instance, 3 mg/100 g vitamin C (see Table 3). Alternatively the term is used when a nutrient is added to a food which does not contain it naturally. In such a case the food is considered as a carrier for that particular nutrient. This is sometimes practised in underdeveloped countries where there is a severe shortage of a particular nutrient (for example, in Guatemala, South America, vitamin A is added to sugar which is a staple food in that country). In Australia the addition of L-ascorbic acid is permitted to foods which do not contain it naturally, such as white and wholemeal flour for making bread. In this case ascorbic acid is used as a bread-improver because it enhances dough performance, but it is destroyed in the processing.

5.4 USE OF L-ASCORBIC ACID AS AN ANTIOXIDANT IN FOODS

An antioxidant is a substance which is capable of retarding or preventing development of oxidative rancidity in food. The antioxidant, that is, the reducing property of L-ascorbic acid, is exploited for the preservation of flavour, colour and appearance of certain foods. In Australia the use of L-ascorbic acid as antioxidant (not as a vitamin) is permitted in meat products such as corned, pickled, salted meat, cooked manufactured meat, in frozen fish (not more than 400 ppm = 40 mg/100 g), in frozen cooked prawns or shrimps (not more than 400 ppm), in dried instant potatoes (not more than 0.01% = 10 mg/100 g) and it may be used during the manufacture of wine. No claim can be made as to the presence in these foods of L-ascorbic acid as a vitamin (Pure Food Act of New South Wales, 1977). Nevertheless some residual vitamin C may be detected by analysing these products (Nobile and Woodhill, 1973; Nobile, Woodhill and Rosevear, 1975, 1976) and this may make a small contribution to the vitamin C content of the diet. Unfortunately the isomer (epimer) of L-ascorbic acid, the erythorbic acid (D-araboascorbic acid or isoascorbic acid), is also a permitted antioxidant for use in Australian foods. This substance has only 1/20 of the vitamin C activity, and may be (and is frequently) used in all the products listed because it is cheaper than L-ascorbic acid. Residual quantities of this substance may be present in some of the foods. As it reacts like L-ascorbic acid with the reagent commonly used for the assay of vitamin C, it is essential to use a special technique (thin layer chromatography) to differentiate between the two substances whenever any of the foods listed above is analysed for vitamin C. If the food contains erythorbic acid its vitamin C content is to be considered nil (Nobile and Woodhill, 1973).

5.5 ASSESSMENT OF FOOD INTAKE FOR VITAMIN C (see Table 3 with explanatory notes)

Today's food supply is highly processed because the modern life-

Table 3 Vitamin C food table[a]

No.[b]	*Food group*[c]*: food*	*Description*[d]	*Unit*[e]	*Calories/unit*	*Vitamin C/unit mg*[f]	*Vitamin C/unit points*[g]	*Reference code*[h]
	Beverages–alcoholic[i]						
1000	Wine	Claret	100 ml	68	0	0	A, B
1001		Rosé	100 ml	71	8.7	0.5	A, B
1002		Moselle	100 ml	66	8.7	0.5	A, B
1003		White, sparkling	100 ml	76	7.3	0.5	A, B
1004		British figures	100 ml	75 (68–94)	0	0	B
1005		US figures	100 ml	75 (68–94)	(–)	(–)	B, C
1006		Port	100 ml	157	0	0	B
1007		Sherry, dry	100 ml	116	0	0	B
1008		sweet	100 ml	136	0	0	B
	Beverages – non-alcoholic						
1009	Carbonated[j]	Cola type, gingerale, lemonade, orange	300 ml	132	0	0	A, B, C, D
1010	Cordials[j]	diluted 1:4, various flavours: lemon, lime, orange	300 ml	84	0	0	A, B, C, D
	Fruit juices						
1011	Grapefuit	canned, unsweetened, 10 cans, 7 brands	100 ml	31	28	2	B
1012		canned, unsweetened, 10 cans, 7 brands	300 ml	93	84	5.5	B
1013		canned, sweetened, 5 cans of different brands	100 ml	38	29	2	B
1014		canned, sweetened, 5 cans of different brands	300 ml	114	87	6	B
1015	Orange	canned, unsweetened, 9 cans, 6 brands	100 ml	33	35	2.5	B
1016		canned, unsweetened, 9 cans, 6 brands	300 ml	99	105	7	B

No.[b]	Food group[c]: food	Description[d]	Unit[e]	Calories/unit	Vitamin C/unit mg[f]	Vitamin C/unit points[g]	Reference code[h]
1017		canned, sweetened, 5 cans, 4 brands	100 ml	51	31	2	B
1018		canned, sweetened, 5 cans, 4 brands	300 ml	153	93	6	B
1019	Pineapple	canned, 6 cans of different brands	100 ml	53	8	0.5	B
1020		canned, 6 cans of different brands	300 ml	159	24	1.5	B
1021	Ribena (blackcurrant)	undiluted, mixed sample	30 ml	69	63	4	B
1022	Rosehip syrup	undiluted, 9 bottles, 4 brands	30 ml	70	88	6	B
1023	Tomato	canned, 10 cans, 6 brands	100 ml	16	20	1.5	B
	Fruit						
1024	Apples[k], eating	flesh only, no skin or core	100 g	46	3		B
1025		Cox's Orange Pippin, flesh only, no skin or core	100 g	46	3		B
1026		unpeeled	100 g	46	5	0.5	B
1027		Golden Delicious, flesh only, no skin or core	100 g	46	3		B
1028		unpeeled	100 g	46	10	0.5	B
1029		Granny Smith, flesh only, no skin or core	100 g	46	2		B
1030		unpeeled	100 g	46	8	0.5	B
1031		Laxton Superb, flesh only, no skin or core	100 g	46	3		B
1032		unpeeled	100 g	46	10	0.5	B
1033		Newton Wonder, flesh only, no skin or core	100 g	46	3		B
1034		unpeeled	100 g	46	10	0.5	B
1035	Apples, cooking	raw, flesh only, no skin or core	100 g	37	15	1	B
1036		Bramley's Seedlings, flesh only, no skin or core	100 g	37	15	1	B
1037		unpeeled	100 g	37	20	1.5	B
1038		Lord Lambourne, flesh only, no skin or core	100 g	37	10	0.5	B
1039		unpeeled	100 g	37	16	1	B

1040		Sturmer Pippin, flesh only, no skin or core	100 g	37	20	1.5	B
1041		unpeeled	100 g	37	30	2	B
1042		Worcester Pearmain, flesh only, no skin or core	100 g	37	10	0.5	B
1043		unpeeled	100 g	37	16	1	B
1044	Apples[l], dried	uncooked	10 g	29	1		D
1045	Apricots	raw, fresh, flesh and skin, no stones	100 g	28	7	0.5	B
1046		stewed with sugar (no stones)	100 g	60	5	0.5	B
1047		canned, fruit and syrup	100 g	106	2		B
1048		dried	100 g	182	trace		B
1049	Avocado pears	Fuerte variety, 10 pears, flesh only	100 g	223	15 (5–30)	1	B
1050	Bananas	flesh only, no skin, 14 samples	100 g	79	8 (6–12)	0.5	A, B
1051		dried	100 g	(–)	0	0	A
1052	Bilberries	raw, whole fruit	100 g	56	22 (10–44)	1.5	B
1053	Blackberries	raw, whole fruit	100 g	29	20	1.5	B
1054		stewed with sugar, fruit and juice	100 g	60	14	1	B
1055	Bush bananas[m]	raw	100 g	(–)	16.7	1	A
1056	Cherries, eating	raw, flesh and skin, no stalks or stones	100 g	47	5	0.5	B
1057	cooking	stewed with sugar, without stones	100 g	77	3		B
1058	Cranberries	raw, whole fruit	100 g	15	12	1	B
1059	Currants, black	whole fruit, no stalks	100 g	28	200 (150–230)	13.5	B
1060		stewed with sugar, fruit and juice	100 g	59	140	9.5	B
1061		canned	100 g	59	100	6.5	B
1062	Currants, red	whole fruit, no stalks	100 g	21	40	2.5	B
1063		stewed with sugar, fruit and juice	100 g	53	28	2	B
1064	Currants, dried	whole fruit	50 g	122	0	0	B
1065	Dates	dried, flesh and skin	50 g	124	0	0	A, B
1066	Figs	green, raw, whole fruit, no skin	100 g	41	2		B
1067		dried, raw	50 g	106	0	0	B

No:[b]	Food group[c]: food	Description[d]	Unit[e]	Calories/unit	Vitamin C/unit mg[f]	Vitamin C/unit points[g]	Reference code[h]
1068	Gooseberries	green, raw, flesh, skin and pips, no tops nor tails	100 g	17	40 (25–50)	2.5	B
1069		stewed with sugar	100 g	50	28	2	B
1070		canned	100 g	50	24	1.5	B
1071		ripe, raw, flesh, skin and pips, no tops nor tails	100 g	37	40 (25–50)	2.5	B
1072	Grapes	black, raw, flesh only, no skin or pips or stalks	100 g	61	4	0.5	B
1073		white, raw, flesh only, no skin or pips or stalks	100 g	63	4	0.5	B
1074	Grapefruit	raw, flesh only, no skin, pith or pips	100 g	22	40 (35–45)	2.5	B
1075		canned, 10 cans, fruit and syrup	100 g	60	30	2	B
1076	Guavas	canned, 10 cans, fruit and syrup	100 g	60	180	12	B
1077	Lemons	whole fruit, including skin, no pips	10 g	2	8	0.5	B
1078		juice, fresh strained from fresh lemons	50 g	4	25 (20–30)	1.5	B
1079	Limes	fresh, whole fruit	10 g	2	2.5		B
1080	Loganberries	raw, whole fruit	100 g	17	35	2.5	B
1081		stewed with sugar, fruit and juice	100 g	54	26	1.5	B
1082		canned, fruit and juice	100 g	101	25	1.5	B
1083	Lychees	raw, flesh only, literature sources	100 g	64	40	2.5	B
1084		canned, 10 cans, fruit and syrup	100 g	68	8	0.5	B
1085	Mandarins	raw, peeled, 3 samples	100 g	46	14 (13–15)	1	A, D
1086		canned, 10 cans, fruit and syrup	100 g	56	14	1	B
1087	Mangoes	raw, flesh only: literature sources	100 g	59	30 (10–180)	2	A, B

1088		canned, 10 cans, fruit and syrup	100 g	77	10	0.5	B
1089	Melons, Cantaloupe	raw, flesh only, no skin or seeds	100 g	24	25	1.5	B
1090	Yellow honey-dew	raw, flesh only, no skin or seeds	100 g	21	25	1.5	B
1091	Watermelon	raw, flesh only, no skin or seeds	100 g	21	5	0.5	B
1092	Mulberries	raw, whole fruit	100 g	36	10	0.5	B
1093	Nectarines	raw, flesh, and skin, no stones	100 g	50	(8)	0.5	B
1094	Olives	all types: black, green, bottled	50 g	52	0	0	A, B
1095	Oranges	raw, flesh only, no peel or pips	100 g	35	50 (40–60)	3.5	B
1096		juice, fresh strained from fresh oranges, also frozen, reconstituted orange juice	100 g	38	50 (40–60)	3.5	B
1097	Passion fruit	Granadilla, raw, flesh and seeds, no skin	50 g	17	10	0.5	B
1098	Paw paw (papaya)	raw, edible portion	100 g	41	64	4.5	C, D
1099		raw, edible portion, cubed	100 g	41	55	3.5	C, D
1100		canned, 10 cans, fruit and juice	100 g	65	15	1	B
1101	Peaches	fresh, raw, flesh and skin, no stones	100 g	37	8	0.5	B
1102		canned, sweetened, sliced	100 g	87	0–1		A,B
1103		dried, whole fruit, raw	100 g	212	trace		B
1104	Pears, eating	raw, flesh only, no skin or core	100 g	41	3		A, B
1105	cooking	raw, flesh only, no skin or core	100 g	36	3		B
1106		stewed with sugar, flesh and juice, peeled and cored before cooking	100 g	65	2		B
1107		canned, fruit and syrup	100 g	77	1		B
1108	Pineapple	fresh, flesh only, no skin or core	100 g	46	25 (20–40)	1.5	B
1109		canned, fruit and syrup	100 g	77	12	1	B
1110	Plums[n]	raw, flesh and skin, no stones or stalks	100 g	38	3		B
1111	cooking	stewed with sugar, fruit and juice, no stones	100 g	59	2		B
1112	Pomegranates	juice from fresh fruit	100 g	44	8	0.5	B
1113	Prunes	dried, raw, flesh and skin, no stones	100 g	161	0–trace		A, B

No:[b]	Food group[c]: food	Description[d]	Unit[e]	Calories/unit	Vitamin C/unit mg[f]	Vitamin C/unit points[g]	Reference code[h]
1114	Quinces	raw, flesh, no skin or core	100 g	25	15	1	B
1115	Raisins	dried, flesh and skin, no stones	100 g	246	0	0	B
1116		wild[o]	30 g	(–)	17	1	A
1117	Raspberries	whole fruit, fresh	50 g	12	13 (7–18)	1	B
1118		whole fruit, frozen	50 g	3	10	0.5	B
1119		stewed with sugar, fruit and juice	50 g	34	11	0.5	B
1120		canned, fruit and syrup	50 g	44	4	0.5	B
1121	Rhubarb	stewed with sugar, stems and juice	100 g	45	7	0.5	B
1122		canned	100 g	45	1		B
1123	Strawberries	raw, flesh and pips, no stalks	100 g	26	60 (40–90)	4	B
1124		frozen	100 g	26	50	3.5	B
1125		canned, 10 cans, fruit and syrup	100 g	81	21	1.5	B
1126	Sultanas	dried, whole fruit	50 g	125	0	0	B
1127	Tangerines	raw, flesh only, no peel or pips	100 g	34	30	2	B
	Vegetables[p]						
1128	Ackee	canned, 8 cans, drained contents only	100 g	151	30	2	B
1129	Artichokes	globe, base of leaves and soft inside parts: boiled 35 minutes	100 g	15	3		B
1130		Jerusalem, flesh only; boiled 20 minutes	100 g	18	2		B
1131	Asparagus[q]	soft tips only; boiled 25 minutes	100 g	18	20 (15–30)	1.5	B
1132		canned, green	100 g	18	15	1	A, D
1133	Aubergine (eggplant)	baked	100 g	62	3		D
1134	Beans, french	pods and beans cut up; boiled 30 minutes	100 g	7	5	0.5	B
1135	runner	trimmed, pods broken up; boiled 20 minutes	100 g	19	5	0.5	B

1136		canned	100 g	19	2		B
1137	broad	whole beans, without pods; boiled 30 minutes	100 g	48	15	1	B
1138		canned	100 g	48	6	0.5	B
1139	dried	various types, soaked 24 hours; boiled 2 hours	100 g	93	0	0	B
1140	Bean sprouts[q]	fresh	100 g	9	30	2	B
1141		canned, 10 cans, drained contents	100 g	9	1		B
1142	Beetroot	flesh only, no skin: boiled 2 hours, weighed cold	100 g	44	5	0.5	B
1143	Broccoli[q]	raw, 10 samples, predominantly leaves, thick stems removed	100 g	23	110 (70–160)	7.5	B
1144		cooked, 10 samples, predominantly leaves, thick stems removed; boiled 15 minutes	100 g	18	34 (20–70)	2.5	B
1145	Brussels sprouts[q]	raw, 10 samples, inner leaves only	100 g	26	90 (70–140)	6	B
1146		cooked, 10 samples, inner leaves only; boiled 15 minutes	100 g	18	40 (30–90)	2.5	B
1147	Cabbage, red	raw, inner leaves	100 g	20	55	3.5	B
1148	Savoy	raw, inner leaves	100 g	26	60 (50–80)	4	B
1149		cooked, inner leaves; boiled 30 minutes	100 g	9	15 (10–40)	1	B
1150	spring	inner leaves; boiled 30 minutes	100 g	7	25 (10–50)	1.5	B
1151	white	raw, 7 cabbages, whole as purchased	100 g	22	40	2.5	B
1152		shredded	100 g	22	32	2	B
1153	winter	January King, raw, 20 cabbages, inner leaves	100 g	22	55 (40–70)	3.5	B
1154		January King, cooked, inner leaves; boiled 20 minutes	100 g	15	20 (10–40)	1.5	B

No.[b]	Food group[c]: food	Description[d]	Unit[e]	Calories/unit	Vitamin C/unit mg[f]	Vitamin C/unit points[g]	Reference code[h]
1155	Carrots, old	raw, flesh only	100 g	23	6 (4–10)	0.5	B
1156		cooked, flesh only, cut up; boiled 45 minutes	100 g	19	4 (2–6)	0.5	B
1157	Carrots, young	purchased with leaves, flesh only; boiled 25 minutes	100 g	20	4 (2–6)	0.5	B
1158		canned, 6 samples, drained contents	100 g	19	3		B
1159	Cauliflower[q]	raw, 16 cauliflowers, flowers and stalk	100 g	13	60 (50–90)	4	B
1160		cooked, 16 cauliflowers, flowers and stalk; boiled 20 minutes	100 g	9	20 (15–40)	1.5	B
1161	Celeriac	flesh only; boiled 30 minutes	100 g	14	4	0.5	B
1162	Celery	raw, stems only	100 g	8	7	0.5	B
1163		cooked, stems only; boiled 30 minutes	100 g	5	5	0.5	B
1164	Chicory	raw, stems and young leaves	100 g	9	4	0.5	B
	Courgettes (see Zucchini)						
1165	Cucumber	raw, flesh only	50 g	5	4	0.5	B
1166	Endive	raw, leaves only	10 g	2	1.5		B
1167	Horseradish	raw, flesh of roots	5 g	3	6	0.5	B
1168	Leeks	raw, bulb only	100 g	31	18 (15–30)	1	B
1169		cooked, bulb only; boiled 30 minutes	100 g	24	15 (10–25)	1	B
1170	Lentils	dried, as purchased	100 g	304	trace		B
1171	Lettuce	raw, 29 lettuces, inner leaves of long and headed forms	10 g	2	1.5 (1–3)		B

1172	Marrow	flesh only; boiled 25 minutes	100 g	7	2		B
1173	Mushrooms	raw, flesh and stems	50 g	6	1.5		B
1174		cooked: flesh and stems; fried in dripping (fat)	50 g	105	0.5		B
1175	Mustard and cress	raw, leaves and stems	10 g	1	4	0.5	B
1176	Okra (ladies' fingers)	raw, literature sources	50 g	8	12	1	B
1177	Onions	raw, flesh only	50 g	12	5 (1.5–7.5)	0.5	B
1178		cooked, flesh only; boiled 30 minutes	100 g	13	6	0.5	B
1179		cooked, flesh only, cut up; fried in margarine, 3 samples	100 g	345	5 (1–8)	0.5	A, B
1180	Onion, spring	raw, flesh of bulbs	10 g	4	2.5 (2–3)		B
1181	Parsley	raw, leaves	10 g	2	15 (10–20)	1	B
1182		dried, flakes, bottled	5 g	(–)	17.5	1	A
1183	Parsnips	flesh only; boiled 30 minutes	100 g	56	10 (5–20)	0.5	B
1184	Peas, fresh	whole peas, no pods; boiled 20 minutes	100 g	52	15	1	B
1185	frozen	15 packets, boiled 5 minutes	100 g	41	13	1	B
1186	air-dried	cooked	100 g	52	11	0.5	B
1187	freeze-dired	cooked	100 g	52	16	1	B
1188	garden	canned, 10 cans, drained contents	100 g	47	8	0.5	B
1189	processed	canned, 10 cans, drained contents	100 g	80	trace		B
1190	dried	raw, various types: split, chick, etc.,	100 g	286	trace		B
1191		cooked, various types: split, chick, etc., soaked 24 hours; boiled 2 hours	100 g	103	trace		B
1192	Peppers, green	raw, 30 peppers, flesh only	10 g	2	10 (6–17)	0.5	B
1193		cooked, 30 peppers, flesh only; boiled 15 minutes	100 g	14	60	4	B
1194	Plantain, green	10 samples: boiled 30 minutes	100 g	122	3		B

No.[b]	Food group[c]:food	Description[d]	Unit[e]	Calories/unit	Vitamin C/unit mg[f]	Vitamin C/unit points[g]	Reference code[h]
1195	Potatoes[r], new	boiled 15 minutes, flesh only	100 g	76	18	1	B
1196		canned, 10 cans, drained contents	100 g	53	17	1	B
1197	old, fresh	baked in skins, flesh only	100 g	85	5–16	0.5–1	B
1198		boiled 30 minutes, flesh only	100 g	80	4–14	0.5–1	B
1199		boiled 15–35 minutes, flesh only, 18 samples	100 g	80	4–11	0.5–1	A, B
1200		boiled and mashed with margarine and milk	100 g	119	4–12	0.5–1	B
1201		chips: fried in deep fat	100 g	253	5–16	0.5–1	B
1202		roasted in shallow fat, flesh only	100 g	157	5–16	0.5–1	B
1203	old, frozen	11 packets as purchased	100 g	109	6	0.5	B
1204		11 packets as purchased; fried in shallow fat	100 g	291	4	0.5	B
1205	Potatoes, crisps	26 packets, mixed plain and flavoured	10 g	53	1.7		B
1206	Potato powder[s], instant	20 packets, made up, calculated from the powder	100 g	70	3		B
1207	Pumpkin	baked 40 minutes in lamb dripping (fat)	100 g	130	6	0.5	A, D
1208		boiled 20 minutes	100 g	31	7	0.5	A, D
1209		steamed 7 minutes in pressure cooker	100 g	31	5	0.5	A, D
1210	Radishes	raw, flesh and skins	50 g	8	12.5 (5–17.5)	1	B
1211	Salsify	boiled 45 minutes, flesh only	100 g	18	4	0.5	B
1212	Seakale	boiled 20 minutes, stems only	100 g	8	18	1	B
1213	Silverbeet	boiled 10–40 minutes, leaves only, 3 samples	100 g	30	1–4	0.5	A, D
1214	Spinach	leaves, boiled 15 minutes without added water	100 g	30	25 (10–60)	1.5	B
1215	Spring greens	leaves, boiled 30 minutes	100 g	10	30 (20–70)	2	B

1216	Swedes	raw, flesh only	100 g	21	25 (15–40)	1.5	B
1217		cooked, flesh only, boiled 45 minutes	100 g	18	17 (8–25)	1	B
1218	Sweet corn, on-the-cob	16 cobs, kernels only, boiled 15 minutes	100 g	123	9	0.5	B
1219	Sweet corn	canned kernels, 10 cans, whole contents	100 g	76	5	0.5	B
1220	Sweet potatoes	boiled 30 minutes, flesh only	100 g	85	15	1	B
1221	Tomatoes	raw, flesh, skin and seeds	100 g	14	20 (10–30)	1.5	B
1222		cooked, flesh, skin and seeds: fried in dripping (fat), 6 samples	100 g	69	5–11	0.5	A, B
1223		canned, 10 cans, drained contents	100 g	12	18	1	B
1224	Turnips, white	raw, flesh only	100 g	20	25 (15–40)	1.5	B
1225		cooked, flesh only; boiled 30 minutes	100 g	14	17 (8–25)	1	B
1226	Turnip tops	leaves, boiled 20 minutes	100 g	11	40 (20–70)	2.5	B
1227	Watercress	raw, leaves and part of stems	10 g	1	6 (4–8)	0.5	B
1228	Yam	flesh only: boiled 30 minutes, 6 samples	100 g	119	2		B
1229	Zucchini (courgettes)	cut in rings: boiled 4 minutes	100 g	(–)	7	0.5	A
1230		cut in rings: fried 15 minutes in butter	100 g	(–)	8	0.5	A
	Offal'						
1231	Brains, calf	soaked 2 hours, boiled 35 minutes, 5 samples	100 g	152	17	1	B
1232	lamb	soaked 2 hours: boiled 20 minutes, 11 samples	100 g	126	17	1	B
1233	calf and sheep	crumbed and fried	100 g	291	13	1	D
1234	Heart, sheep	roasted, ventricles only	100 g	237	(11)	1	B
1235	ox	stewed, fat and valves removed before cooking, 18 samples	100 g	179	6	0.5	B

No[b].	Food group[c]:food	Description[d]	Unit[e]	Calories/unit	Vitamin C/unit mg[f]	Vitamin C/unit points[g]	Reference code[h]
1236	Kidneys, lamb	fried, core removed before cooking, 19 samples	100 g	155	9	0.5	B
1237	ox	stewed, core removed before cooking, 18 samples	100 g	172	10	0.5	B
1238	pig	stewed, core removed before cooking, 20 samples	100 g	153	11	0.5	B
1239	Liver, calf	fried, coated in seasoned flour, 12 samples	100 g	254	13	1	B
1240	chicken	fried, coated in seasoned flour, 16 samples	100 g	194	13	1	B
1241	lamb	fried, coated in seasoned flour, 18 samples	100 g	232	12	1	B
1242	ox	stewed, coated in seasoned flour, 18 samples	100 g	198	15	1	B
1243	pig	stewed, coated in seasoned flour, 18 samples	100 g	189	9	0.5	B
1244	Sweetbread, lamb	soaked 2 hours, boiled 1 hour, then coated with egg and bread crumbs, fried	100 g	230	18	1	B
1245	Tongue, sheep	stewed, fat and skin removed	100 g	289	(6)	0.5	B
1246	ox	boiled, fat and skin removed	100 g	293	(2)		B
1247	Tripe	stewed in milk, lime treated before purchase, 18 samples	100 g	100	(3)		B
	Fish						
1248	Roe[u], cod	hard, raw, literature sources	50 g	56	15	1	B
1249		parboiled, sliced, crumbed, fried	50 g	101	(13)	1	B
1250	herring	soft, raw, literature sources	50 g	40	2.5		B
1251		rolled in flour, fried	50 g	122	(2.5)		B
	Milks[v]						
1252	Milk, cows'	pasteurized, homogenized, literature sources, Milk Marketing Board	100 g	65	0.5–7		B

1253		boiled	100 g	65	0–1		B
1254		sterilized	100 g	65	0–1		B
1255		dried, skimmed, 10 tins, 4 different brands	100 g	355	6	0.5	B
1256		dried, whole, mixed samples, 3 different types	100 g	490	10	0.5	B
1257	goats'	literature sources	100 g	71	1.5		B
1258	human	mixed samples from 96 mothers about 1 month postpartum	100 g	69	3.7		B
	Jams[w] and marmalades						
1259	Jam, blackcurrant		50 g	130	12	1	B
1260	mixed berries	blackberry, blackcurrant, gooseberry, raspberry, strawberry, fruit with edible seeds, 2 samples of each, different brands	50 g	130	5	0.5	B
1261	mixed stonefruit	apricot, damson, greengage, plum, 2 samples of each, different brands	50 g	130	trace		B
1262	Marmalade	4 brands	50 g	130	5	0.5	B
	Tomato products						
1263	Tomato, *purée*[x]	*purée* or paste in tubes, calculated value	10 g	07	(10)	0.5	B
1264	sauce	6 bottles, different brands	10 g	10	1		B, D

EXPLANATORY NOTES FOR TABLE 3

[a] Table 3 is designed to:

(1) provide a ready-reckoner for the vitamin C content of specified units of foods showing their contribution to the vitamin C content of the diet, and so
(2) enable a food intake to be assessed for its vitamin C content.

Preferred figures have been used for some of the items. The word 'preferred' can be defined as the mode, in other words, the most frequently occurring or the most fashionable. The preferred figure is not the arithmetic mean or the average. A preferred figure has to be chosen if only a few analysed values are available and the range of values is very wide. On the other hand, if data from a large number of food samples are available, a single extreme value would have little effect on the average or the mean; a judgement by the food table compilers would not have to be exercised and the arithmetic mean could be used.

The term *selected value* is used by compilers of food tables (Paul and Southgate, 1978). This is a general term similar to preferred values and means the selection of values after critical assessment of the values reported in the literature. Consideration is given to the nature and origin of the samples, cooking, preparation and analytical methods. All values in Table 3 are expressed as *edible portions*, that is, the part of the food which can be eaten. Values are given for some foods such as apples with or without skins because sometimes the skins are eaten and sometimes discarded.

Which food items should be included in a vitamin C food table? Not only are the rich sources of vitamin C listed in Table 3, but also foods that have a *low* vitamin C content. If these poor sources of vitamin C are eaten in large quantities their vitamin C contribution to the diet becomes significant. Foods such as meat and cereals that are known to make no contribution to the vitamin C content of the diet have not been included. Some types of meat products, such as brains, liver and kidneys were found to retain vitamin C in the cooked state. These items have been included as they may be^ome important sources of vitamin C if consumed in quantity, and the data on their vitamin C content would be essential for dietary assessment. Some food items which have nil vitamin C content have also been included in the table to point up the contrast between certain foods. Unusual sources of vitamin C have been included and their significance in the food pattern are discussed in the explanatory notes below. Ranges of vitamin C are given in parentheses for some foods which are important sources of the vitamin; these ranges can help the diet assessor understand the confidence which should be given to the values for vitamin C for a particular intake of food.

[b] The number assigned to the food item commences with 1000 and all items have a four-digit coding number which serves to identify the foods.

[c] In food composition tables the foods are usually divided into groups and listed alphabetically. This is a practical way of classification and is related to meal pattern and menu planning. Table 3 itself is a grouping of foods based on their contribution to the vitamin C content of the diet and is not in alphabetical order. However, the foods within each group have been listed in alphabetical order according to the most commonly used name for the food. All foods in Table 3 appear in the index of this book. This listing of food groups is:

Beverages
Fruit
Vegetables
Offal
Fish roe
Milk
Jams and marmalade
Tomato products

The following conventional symbols of Food Composition Tables have been used:

0 in the table signifies that virtually no vitamin C is known to be present in the food.

( ) 'Figures in parentheses are estimates taken from related foods or, more rarely, tentative values based on a limited number of published sources' (Paul and Southgate, 1978). Ranges of values are also given in parentheses.

(–) shows that no information is available, either from direct analysis or from the literature. This does *not* signify that the food does not contain vitamin C.

[d] The description of the food in detail is of great value when substitutions have to be made, if the particular item required for a dietary assessment is not given in the tables.
[e] Units have been used rather than the terms 'portion or serving' and the units are defined for each food item. The sizes of the units are chosen to correspond with an appropriate measure used in the meal pattern. For instance, orange juice is usually consumed in either a small glass (100 ml capacity) or a large glass (300 ml capacity), so both units are given for orange juice with their corresponding vitamin C content. This simplifies calculation of the vitamin C content of a diet. For most of the items 100 g is a convenient portion size and makes calculation easy. In vegetables occasionally a smaller unit is used where a 100 g serving is considered too large. In some cases the unit of 100 g has been given to allow easy comparison between the raw and cooked vegetable. For the purpose of this table we considered 100 ml of alcoholic and non-alcoholic beverages approximately equal to 100 g.
[f] The vitamin C content is listed in milligrams (mg) per unit. This differs from tables that give the vitamin C composition in milligrams per 100 g weight of every food. In the table either a single figure is given or, if the range of values is known to be wide in a particular food, the width of the range is indicated.
[g] Vitamin C points per unit of food are given in this column. The originator of this method of dietary assessment for all nutrients was Stucky (1979). The points are often called Stucky points but for simplicity we will refer to them simply as points. One point for vitamin C is 15 mg which is midway between 11 mg and 19 mg. For dietary assessment this limited accuracy is acceptable. When rating a diet for any nutrient (such as vitamin C) a quantitative measure is needed for comparison with a yardstick of nutritional adequacy. This procedure is an improvement upon the method of dietary assessment which indicates that a food is an excellent, good or very poor source of a nutrient. The point system has become a quantitative measure for nutrition education to replace the qualitative vague instructions included in the Good Food Source Method or the Food Group and Exchange List Methods. The points are rounded off to 0.5 (for instance, $\pm$ 0.25) of a point. If a significant quantity of a food with less vitamin C than 0.5 points per unit has been eaten, the milligrams in the adjacent column can be added up and the total milligrams per day can be divided by 15 to give the total points per day. The point-notation for the vitamin C content of packaged foods could be used for food labelling. It would be educational and much simpler than relating the nutrient content of a package to a certain percentage of the dietary allowance as is currently done voluntarily by food manufacturers in the United States.
[h] The capital letters A, B, C, and D in this column are the coded reference source for each item. Each letter refers to a group of references: A from Australian analysed values, B from the United Kingdom, C from the United States, and D from the Food Composition Table of Australia. These references are all included individually in the general reference list of the book, which is arranged alphabetically according to the author's name, and also given below for ease of reference and to make the table complete.

A = Nobile, S. and Woodhill, J.M. (1973). A survey of the vitamin content of some 2000 foods as they are consumed by selected groups of the Australian population. *Food Technol. Aust.*, **25(2)**, 80
Nobile, S., Woodhill, J.M. and Rosevear, P.E. (1975). A survey of the vitamin content of foods as they are consumed by selected groups of the Australian population. *Food Technol. Aust.*, **27(9)**, 342
Nobile, S., Woodhill, J. M. and Rosevear, P.E. (1976). A survey of the vitamin content of foods as they are consumed by selected groups of the Australian population. *Food Technol. Aust.*, **28(11)**, 427

B = Paul, A.A. and Southgate, D.A.T. (1978). *McCance and Widdowson's The Composition of Foods*. 4th revised and extended edition of Medical Research Council's Special Report No. 297. (London: HMSO)

C = Watt, B.K. and Merrill A.L. (1963). *Composition of Foods, Raw, Processed, Prepared*. Agriculture Handbook No. 8. (Washington, DC: Agricultural Services, US Department of Agriculture)

D = Thomas, S. and Corden, M. (1970), (1977). *Tables of Composition of Australian Foods*. (Canberra: Australian Government Publishing Service)

[i] Some samples of beer and wine have been found on analysis to contain vitamin C. The addition of L-ascorbic acid to these beverages is permitted by law (Pure Food Act of New South Wales, 1977) but no claim can be made. Only traces of vitamin C were found in some samples of beer which would not make a contribution if drunk in normal amounts (300 ml). These data are not included. The samples of wine as reported would provide 7–9 mg vitamin C per 100 ml or per unit. Other types of spirits are not included in the table because they do not contain any vitamin C.
[j] L-Ascorbic acid may be added to some brands. There is loss on storage of open bottles particularly when exposed to light.
[k] There is variation in the vitamin C content of apples; storage and environment are factors. Unpeeled apples have more vitamin C than peeled ones.
[l] Dried apples lose their vitamin C content on cooking.
[m] A bush fruit eaten by Australian Aborigines; it grows near Alice Springs and its botanical name is *Leichhardtia australis* R.Br.
[n] Including damsons.
[o] Bush fruit eaten by Aborigines and growing in Alice Springs, its botanical name is *Solanum centrale*, J.M. Black.
[p] The vitamin C content of vegetables is very variable and depends upon the treatment of the vegetable; freshness and correct storage is important, and bruising and shredding destroys vitamin C. Cooking losses are dependent upon the length of time and the amount of water used. Vitamin C leaches out into the cooking water particularly if any softening agent, such as bicarbonate of soda, has been added. Air-drying of vegetables usually destroys vitamin C.
[q] Vitamin C is in growing points hence the high concentration in asparagus, bean sprouts, broccoli, brussels sprouts and cauliflower.
[r] See Table 2 for losses of vitamin C occurring during storage of raw potatoes, and cooking of potatoes by various methods.
[s] Some brands of potato powder are fortified with ascorbic acid and may contain up to ten times these values.
[t] Meat is not a good source of vitamin C but the vitamin is present in active metabolic tissues; so it is to be expected that brains, liver, sweetbreads and to a certain extent heart, kidneys and tongue would be a rich source of vitamin C. Some brands of canned meat, such as ham, ham and pork chopped, and luncheon meat, may sometimes contain L-ascorbic acid – from 12 to 60 mg/100 g – which is added as an antioxidant (Paul and Southgate, 1978). In Australia (Pure Food Act of New South Wales, 1977) it is permitted to add not more than 40 mg L-ascorbic acid per 100 g meat products, such as corned, pickled, salted meat and cooked manufactured meat. The addition of the biologically inactive optical isomer (epimer), the iso-ascorbic acid or erythorbic acid, is equally permitted. The presence of either L-ascorbic acid or erythorbic acid in these products should be determined by analysis; if erythorbic acid is found the vitamin C content of these products can be considered nil (Nobile and Woodhill, 1973).
[u] The hard roe would have a very low water content, so the vitamin C would be concentrated.
[v] Milk is not considered a good source of vitamin C although human milk contains enough for the baby in the first months of life. Cows' and goats' milk have 1.5 mg vitamin C/100 g if raw and fresh. This falls to 1.0 mg after 12 hours and to 0.5 mg after 24 hours. The vitamin C is concentrated in the dried products.
[w] It is worthwhile eating blackcurrant jam and marmalade for their vitamin C value.
[x] Even 10 g of tomato *purée* makes a worthwhile contribution to the vitamin C content of the diet.

style requires handling and storing of food after harvesting. The shelf-life and keeping qualities are improved by many technological procedures. Vitamin C is one of the essential nutrients which must be included in the daily diet and which is likely to be a casualty. Every little bit counts, and all ways to protect food against losses of vitamin C should be studied in detail.

Assessment of the intake of a nutrient implies estimation, appraisal and the process of assigning a value to the nutrient in the food eaten. The market place offers a wide choice of convenience foods which have been developed to cater for the pace of modern living and the need for ease in food preparation and food service. Two basic tools which have been developed to assist the dietitian-nutritionist in the task of dietary assessment are *tables of food composition*, and the yardstick for nutritional assessment – the *dietary allowances*. Both these tools have limitations and both must be used with discretion based on a knowledge of how the tools were compiled; good judgement must be used (Woodhill, 1951). The dietary allowance yardstick is the crux of how much vitamin C is needed; it is discussed in Chapter 8. Without these two tools not even a rough estimate of the nutritional value of a diet can be made.

Food tables and food analyses usually report the content of nutrients per 100 g portions of the food; this can be troublesome to a person unfamiliar with the portion sizes commonly used, so a unit size portion for each food must be established. Table 3 provides a ready-reckoner for the vitamin C content of the diet. The table includes not only rich but also poor sources of vitamin C – if the latter foods are eaten in large quantities they make a significant contribution to the vitamin C content of the diet. In Table 3 data are reported on beverages, fruit, vegetables, offal, milk, jams and tomato products as eaten. Extensive explanatory notes accompany the table.

5.6 WHY FOOD IN PREFERENCE TO ASCORBIC ACID TABLETS OR CRYSTALLINE ASCORBIC ACID?

It is unwise to cook food carelessly and try to compensate for the losses by taking ascorbic acid tablets. There are other essential nutrients in food that would be destroyed by poor cooking practices and ascorbic acid tablets or crystalline ascorbic acid contain only the one substance: ascorbic acid. It is much better to take it as food rather than tablets because in foods it is present as vitamin C (the redox-system), and there are other essential nutrients in food. For example, flavoured sugary, yellow-coloured, water-based orange cordial with added ascorbic acid can be classed as an 'empty calorie' food. As long ago as 1959, Jolliffe defined 'empty calories' as

> those sources of body energy that are devoid, or nearly so, of essential amino acid-containing proteins, essential fatty acids, essential minerals, and vitamins. The principal empty calorie foods are sugar and hydrogenated cooking fats. Alcohol is another example. A dietary substance is considered a full-calorie food when it supplies in some form one ingredient of protein, essential fatty acids, essential mineral, and vitamins in an amount equal to its percentage energy contribution. Full-calorie sources are the muscle and organ tissues, the starch grains and tubers, the watery vegetables and fruits, and the vegetable oils. Thus, in the selection of a balanced diet of nutritionally superior foods the avoidance of empty calories is an important consideration.

In both plant and animal tissues vitamin C has both sides of the redox equation working, but, when ascorbic acid in tablets or crystalline synthetic ascorbic acid is taken, it is the same substance as present in the food but only half of the system. What happens to the balance of the redox-system? For use of ascorbic acid as a thereapeutic agent see Chapter 12.

6
Vitamin C in the human body

6.1 WHERE DOES IT GO?

Absorption from foods

Vitamin C is absorbed rapidly from the food and in a manner similar to that of glucose (Sauberlich, 1975). In humans, the vitamin is absorbed through the mucous membranes of the mouth, the stomach, and the upper part of the small intestine, and hence passes into the bloodstream (Spencer *et al.*, 1963; Wilson, 1974). 'The mechanism of absorption consists of a passive diffusion of the vitamin through the lipoid cell membranes and of an active partition of the vitamin into the cells lining the lumen of the alimentary canal' (Wilson, 1973a).

According to Gehler and Kubler (1970) at least two body pools of vitamin C exist in the human body. The *labile pool,* which is quickly occupied by the vitamin and corresponds to the extracellular volume of the body, and the *stable pool,* which is more slowly occupied and corresponds to the total body water. It is assumed that penetration of ascorbic acid into the second pool is determined by its rate of conversion into dehydroascorbic acid. Each of these pools appear to play a part in the metabolism of vitamin C. The passage of vitamin C from plasma to tissues (leukocytes or white blood cells) was studied by Wilson and Loh (1969a), Loh and Wilson (1970), and Wilson (1973b). The authors demonstrated that 'it undergoes a regular 24-hour *circadian rhythm* during which maximum values of vitamin C occur at 11.58 am in the leukocytes and at 10.35 am in the plasma'. It appears that there is a reversible flow of vitamin C between the plasma and the leukocytes which is partly governed by factors in the plasma (Mohanram and Srikantia, 1967). The presence of adenosine triphosphate (ATP) and oxygen enhances the uptake of the vitamin by the leukocytes from the plasma indicating that an active energy requiring process is involved. The flow of vitamin C from food to the labile and stable pools is sketched in Figure 5.

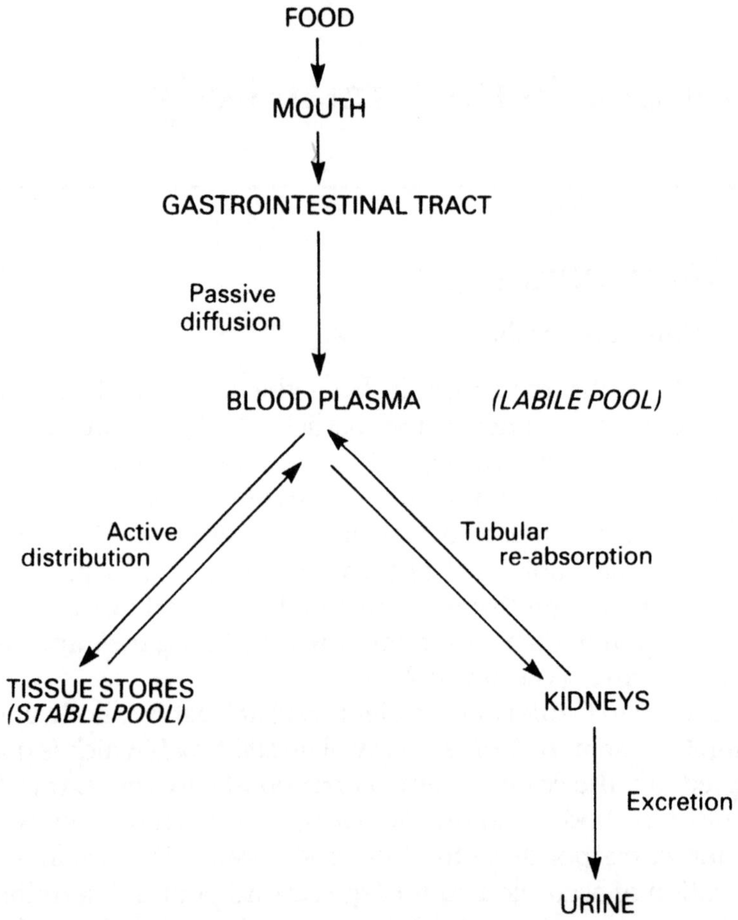

Figure 5 Absorption, distribution, storage and excretion of vitamin C in man. Labile and stable pools

If the quantity of the vitamin which enters the blood after absorption is in excess of tissue saturation, some of it is eliminated rapidly from the kidneys but some is retained in the tissues. Kallner, Hartmann, and Hornig (1977a, b; 1979) reported that intakes of 30 and 60 mg ascorbic acid are absorbed up to 80–90%, and postulated a mean absorption of 70% for intakes up to 180 mg.

When the intake of vitamin C is insufficient to meet metabolic needs, the labile pool is rapidly depleted but depletion of the stable pool is slower. The vitamin is retained in the tissues as long as the cell survives.

Distribution and stores of vitamin C in human tissues and body fluids

In man, as in animals, vitamin C is stored in *tissues* of high metabolic activity. It is most concentrated in the retina and other eye tissues and, in decreasing amounts, in the pituitary gland, corpus luteum, adrenal cortex, thymus, liver, brain, testes, ovaries, spleen, thyroid, pancreas, salivary glands, lungs, kidneys, intestinal wall, heart muscle, spinal fluid, platelets, white blood cells (leukocytes), red blood cells (erythrocytes), and plasma (see Yavorski, Almaden, and King, 1934). The vitamin C content of all these tissues decreases with increasing age. The data in Figure 6 illustrate the decrease of the vitamin C concentration of the pituitary gland, the adrenals, brain, pancreas, thymus, spleen, liver, kidneys and myocardium in post-mortem samples from fetuses, newborns, children, adults and elderly people as reported by Lewin (1976). Most of the data come from studies published in the 1930s. The considerable decrease from birth to old age of the vitamin C content in the brain* first reported by Plaut and Bülow (1935) was confirmed by Schaus (1957). There is a wide range between the results reported by various investigators for the same tissue and in the same age group (see pituitary and adrenal glands in Figure 6). This may be due to individual variations, differences between sexes and/or to differences in the technique used which may have caused losses of the vitamin between time of death and time of assay (Lewin, 1976). It is evident from Table 4 that few or no data are available on the vitamin C content of some *body fluids*. Most investigations have been carried out on the buffy coat (white

* Cerebral cortex: 650 mg to 75 mg; cerebellar cortex: 370 mg to 90 mg; and spinal cord: 160 mg to 110 mg vitamin C per kg wet weight tissue respectively (Schaus, 1957).

blood cells plus platelets), leukocytes (white blood cells), plasma, serum and urine. The values for blood components reported in Table 4 are those considered to approach tissue saturation.

More recent studies (such as Loh and Wilson, 1971b) have indicated that the vitamin C content of blood plasma and white blood cells decreases with increasing age as demonstrated for other human tissues (Figure 6). The difference between ages is seldom taken into account in investigations of population groups. A difference between males and females in the vitamin C content of blood plasma (Woodhill, 1970; 1979; Woodhill and Nobile, 1971a) and white blood cells (Loh and Wilson, 1971c) is known to exist but the issue is controversial and will be discussed in Chapter 9. The *total body pool* of vitamin C, that is, the amount of vitamin C contained in the human body at saturation levels, has been estimated by various methods but the results are conflicting:

(1) 4 to 6 g of vitamin C were found necessary to replenish a person with frank scurvy (Crandon, Lund, and Dill, 1940),
(2) 3 to 4 g of vitamin C were calculated from data on human liver (Lowry, 1952), and
(3) 1.5 g of vitamin C was the average figure found in the four so-called healthy adult male prisoners studied by Baker *et al.* (1969) using labelled ascorbic acid (see Section 6.3).

There seems to be consensus of opinion at least with respect to the total body pool of vitamin C in clinical scurvy. Lowry (1952) reported that it may fall to 200 mg or less and Baker *et al.* (1969) to 300 mg or less. The size of the body pool of vitamin C and its rate of utilization appear to be directly related to the weight of the fat-free body tissue and it has been estimated that approximately 32 to 34 mg of vitamin C are present per kilogram of fat-free body tissue (Sauberlich, 1975). It is said that the vitamin is metabolized, or used up, at a rate of 2–4% (or approximately 3%) of the existing body pool per day (Sauberlich, 1975). This means that an adult individual, to replenish his pool, would require a daily intake of vitamin C of:

(1) 120 to 180 mg, according to Crandon, Lund, and Dill (1940),
(2) 90 to 120 mg, according to Lowry (1952), and
(3) 45 mg average (range 30 to 60 mg), according to Baker *et al.* (1969).

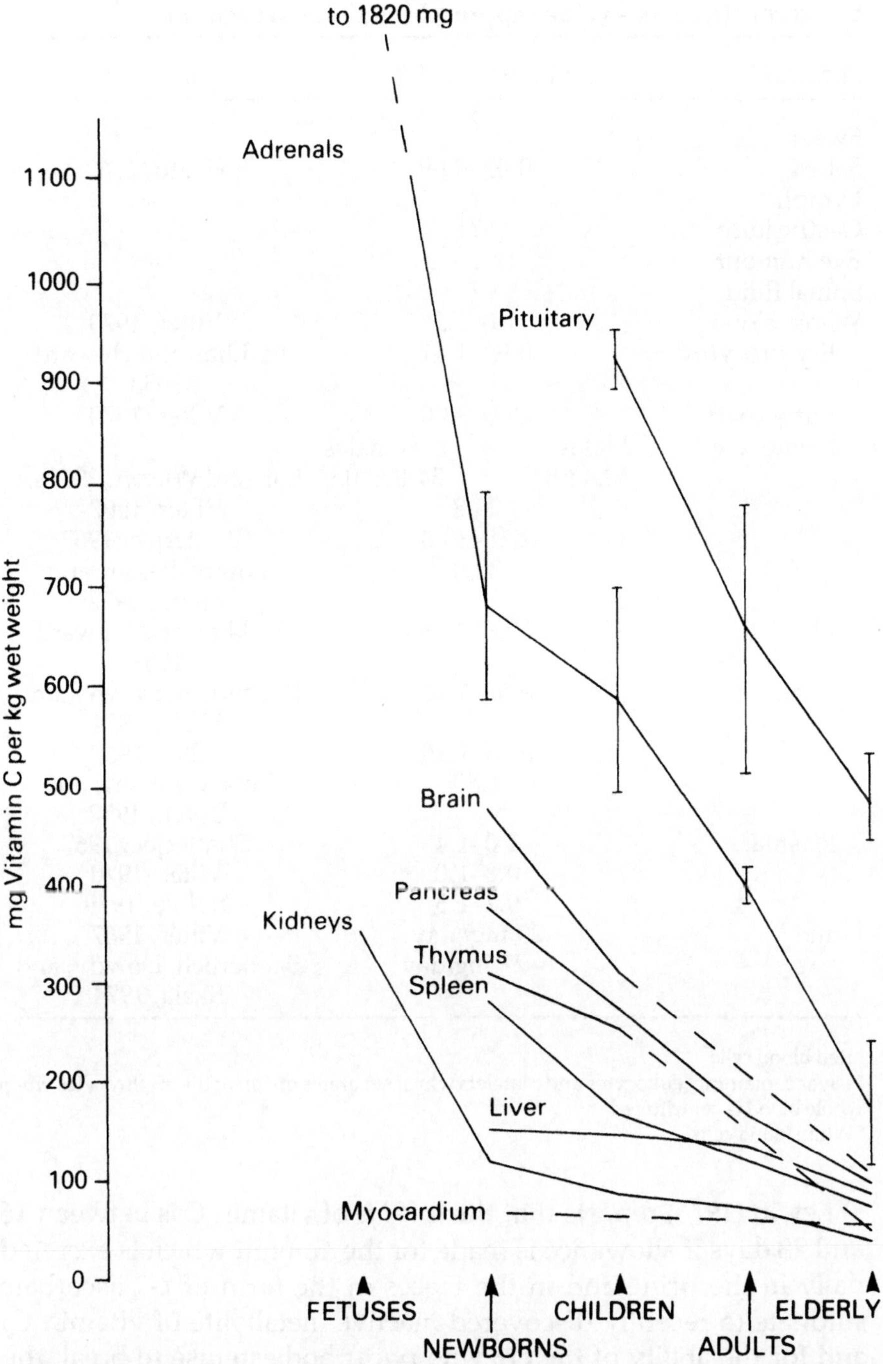

Figure 6 Decrease of the vitamin C content of human tissues with increasing age

Table 4 Vitamin C content in mg/100 ml of human body fluids and blood constituents – values approaching tissue saturation

Body fluid	*mg Vitamin C /100 ml*		*Reference*
Sweat	?		
Saliva	0.07–0.09		Heath, 1962
Lymph	?		–
Gastric juice	?		–
Eye humour	?		–
Spinal fluid	?		–
Whole blood	1.0–1.2		Vilter, 1970
Erythrocytes[a]	0.92–1.41		Barkhan and Howard, 1958
Buffy coat[b]	25.0–38.0		Vilter, 1970
Leukocytes[c]	Males	Females	
	30.4±8.7	34.0±10.9	Loh and Wilson, 1971a,b
	24.2		Vilter, 1967
	27.0–30.0		Chatterjee, 1967
	30.0		Lowry, Bessey and Burch, 1952
Platelets	20.6–32.8		Barkhan and Howard, 1958
Serum	0.69–1.72		Sauberlich, Dowdy, and Skala, 1974
	0.85–1.15		Vilter, 1967
	1.80		Lowry, Bessey, and Burch, 1952
Plasma	1.0–1.4		Chatterjee, 1967
	0.8–1.0		Vilter, 1970
	0.7–1.5		Nobile, 1979
Urine	20 mg/ day		Vilter, 1967
	8–27 mg/day		Sauberlich, Dowdy, and Skala, 1974

[a] Red blood cells
[b] Layer containing leukocytes and platelets which separates on top of the erythrocytes when whole blood is centrifuged
[c] White blood cells

Lewin (1976) reports that the *half-life* of vitamin C is between 16 and 28 days if allowance is made for the amount which is excreted daily in the urine and in the faeces in the form of L-2-ascorbate sulphate (a recently discovered inactive metabolite of vitamin C) and for the ability of the enzyme phosphodiesterase to break the lactone ring of the vitamin C molecule.

Kallner, Hartmann, and Hornig (1977a, b; 1979), using (L-^{14}C) ascorbic acid, studied the time-course of radioactivity in plasma and urine in healthy non-smoking male volunteers under the new approach of 'steady-state conditions' with respect to intake and plasma levels of ascorbic acid. Four doses of dietary intakes were considered: 1 × 30 mg; 2 × 30 mg = 60 mg; 2 × 45 mg = 90 mg; and 4 × 45 mg = 180 mg of crystalline ascorbic acid which was given orally in capsule form. The investigation showed that the overall rate of elimination of ascorbic acid from plasma, the half-life and the size of the body pool appeared to be dose-dependent (Kallner, Hartmann, and Hornig, 1979). The half-life of ascorbic acid was inversely related to the dosage (for example, 40 days on 30 mg intake, 27 days on 60 mg and 13 days on 180 mg). The total body pool was 0.8 g on 30 mg; 1.5 g on 60 mg; and 1.9 g on 180 mg ascorbic acid intake (Kallner, Hartmann, and Hornig, 1977a). The authors concluded that a total turnover of about 60 mg ascorbic acid should be aimed at, but in view of the incomplete absorption of ascorbic acid from foods (Kallner, Hartmann, and Hornig, 1977b) one should ensure a daily intake of 70–75 mg of the vitamin. To extrapolate this figure to 95% of the population an addition of 2 SD or 30 mg ascorbic acid should be considered – a total intake of 100 mg (Kallner, Hartmann, and Hornig, 1979).

Excretion of vitamin C

As vitamin C is very soluble in water it is excreted mainly in the urine where it is found either in the form of ascorbic acid (AA), or as inactive products of vitamin C catabolism. A minimal amount of AA is lost in sweat and in the faeces. The loss in the latter is small – 6–10 mg daily – even when large quantities of vitamin C are taken. Diarrhoea will, however, increase faecal loss.

Excretion in the sweat is said to be low but to increase during physical exercise (Marks, 1968). Vitamin C is mainly excreted in the urine, and the quantity of unaltered ascorbic acid eliminated in this way depends upon intake, body stores and renal function. The plasma threshold value (renal plasma clearance) of vitamin C is just over 1.0 mg/100 ml plasma. At low tubular concentrations in the kidneys about 97–99.5% is reabsorbed (Sigurjonsson, 1951), but traces of ascorbic acid are always present in the urine even at very low plasma levels (Bartley, Krebs, and O'Brien, 1953) and at low intakes (30 mg/day) (Kallner, Hartmann, and Hornig, 1979). This indicates that urinary excretion of intact ascorbic acid does not take place only when the body pool has been saturated. Wide variations between healthy individuals, however, have been found in the amount of ascorbic acid in the urine when high oral doses (700 mg, for example) as used in load tests, were taken (Booth and Todd, 1970).

The quantity and the nature of the *metabolites* of vitamin C also depend upon the amount of the vitamin ingested. At doses of 180 mg or more about 20% of the absorbed ascorbic acid is excreted as metabolites, while that metabolized at low intakes is about 90% (Kallner, Hartmann, and Hornig, 1979). The excretion of intact ascorbic acid decreases rapidly when the intake is inadequate and may fall to trace or zero levels in scurvy. However vitamin C metabolites continue to appear in the urine even when signs and symptoms of scurvy are apparent (Baker *et al.*, 1971). The nature of these metabolites has been extensively studied but so far only a few have been identified (Sauberlich, 1975). Oxalate, traces of dehydro-L-ascorbic acid and diketo-L-gulonic acid have been found as well as derivatives of L-threose and L-threonic acid. The existence of L-2-ascorbate sulphate in the urine has been demonstrated recently, but identification of other stable organic metabolites of vitamin C detected in the urine has not yet been successful (Sauberlich, 1975).

6.2 HOW DOES VITAMIN C FUNCTION?

Partition of the components of the vitamin C redox-system

It is important to know the composition of the vitamin C redox-system in a particular tissue or body fluid in order to understand how vitamin C functions and interacts at the cellular level. Little is known in this respect, but it is known that:

(1) ascorbic acid (AA) – the reduced form of vitamin C – is the main form present in blood plasma and white blood cells (leukocytes), and

(2) dehydroascorbic acid (DHAA) – the oxidized form of vitamin C – is the main form present in the red blood cells (erythrocytes) and in the aqueous humour of the eye when the lens is intact, but when the eye lens is damaged, as in cataract, AA prevails (Müller and Buschke, 1934).

In *vitro* studies have indicated that the white blood cells do not absorb significant amounts of DHAA but simultaneous incubation of red and white blood cells in DHAA results in a significant increase of the AA content of the leukocytes. There seems to be a constant exchange of redox-reactions between white and red blood cells, and iron appears to be involved in the process (Loh and Wilson, 1970).

It is not known in which tissue or body fluid the intermediate component of the vitamin C system, the monodehydroascorbic acid free radical is formed and acts. It is assumed that maintenance of the appropriate relationship between the three forms of vitamin C in a particular body tissue or fluid depends upon its redox-potential, the pH and the concentration of other redox-systems, such as −SH/−S−S-groups. It may also depend upon the rate at which the body receives, absorbs and excretes vitamin C.

Functions known

Studies of vitamin C in the human body commenced soon after the discovery and synthesis of the vitamin, using L-ascorbic acid, because of the more labile nature of dehydro-L-ascorbic acid. It was established in that period that vitamin C:

(1) is essential for the formation and maintenance of the intercellular cement substance, that is, for growth and tissue repair,
(2) has a significant role in the 'safeguarding of the body through the blood', and
(3) plays a part in 'regulating the rate of cellular respiration' (Sherman, 1946).

Further studies demonstrated the correctness of the above findings but the exact mode of action of vitamin C in the human body has not yet been defined. It has been recognized that vitamin C is involved in:

(1) collagen synthesis: in the hydroxylation of proline to hydroxyproline (Peterkofski and Udenfriend, 1965),
(2) amino acid metabolism: conversion of tryptophan to 5-hydroxytryptophan in the pathway of skin melanin (Wagner and Folkers, 1964), and conversion of *p*-hydroxyphenyl pyruvate to homogentisic acid in the formation of tyrosine (Burns, 1961),
(3) synthesis of adrenaline (epinephrine): conversion of 3,4-dihydroxyphenyl alanine to noradrenaline (norepinephrine) which occurs in the adrenal gland (Levin, Levenberg, and Kaufman, 1960) and their protection from oxidation to toxic adrenochromes (Lewin, 1976),
(4) synthesis of anti-inflammatory steroids: formation of hydrocortisone (Burns, 1961) also occurring in the adrenal gland,
(5) reduction of cytochrome *c*, the universal catalyst of cellular respiration (Yamazaki and Piette, 1961),
(6) activation of NADH (nicotinamide adenine dinucleotide reduced) dependent oxidase (Kern and Racker, 1954; Weis, 1975),
(7) protection of the cyclic nucleotides cAMP (cyclic adenosine 3′,5′-monophosphate) and cGMP (cyclic guanosine 3′,5′-monophosphate) from hydrolysis by phosphodiesterase (Lewin, 1976),
(8) iron metabolism: reduction of ferric ions to ferrous ions upon transferral of iron from plasma transferrin to liver transferrin thus enhancing iron absorption (Burns, 1961; Derman *et al.*, 1980),
(9) copper metabolism: maintenance of copper in the reduced form (Scheinberg, 1966), and interaction with copper-containing oxidases and proteins, such as human ceruloplasmin (Dawson, Strothkamp, and Krul, 1975),
(10) Vitamin B_c metabolism: conversion of folic acid to folinic or tetrahydrofolic acid and protection of the same in body stores (Schneider and Staudinger, 1965),
(11) vitamin E synergism during increased metabolic oxidation,

(12) maintenance of –SH-groups such as glutathione at physiological concentrations (Lewin, 1976)
(13) prevention of nitrosamine formation, the carcinogenic substances formed in foods from nitrates (Mirvish, 1975; Raineri and Weisburger, 1975; Lewin, 1976; Newmark and Mergens, 1981).

Further studies indicate that vitamin C may take part in:

(1) metabolism of calcium and of all nutrients involved in growth and bone development (Wohl and Goodhart, 1970),
(2) resistance to toxic components of cigarette smoke (Pelletier, 1968,1970; Ritzel, 1974; Pelletier, 1975; McClean *et al.*, 1976),
(3) prevention of accumulation of histamine in the body (antihistamine effect) (Subramanian *et al.*, 1973),
(4) glucose metabolism (Chatterjee *et al.*, 1975),
(5) detoxication of organochlorine pesticides (Street and Chadwick, 1975),
(6) membrane permeability and interfacial tension (Lewin, 1976).

Interactions and interrelationships of vitamin C with nutrients and metabolites

In summary the functions of vitamin C so far known show that the vitamin interacts with and is interrelated to several essential nutrients and metabolites, for instance:

(1) minerals such as iron, copper and possibly calcium,
(2) vitamins such as vitamin B_c (folic acid), vitamin E, vitamin PP (nicotinamide), possibly vitamin A and vitamin D,
(3) proteins and amino acids,
(4) carbohydrates such as glucose,
(5) fats such as fatty acids,
(6) hormones such as steroid hormones and adrenaline,
(7) cyclic nucleotides such as cyclic AMP (cAMP) and cyclic GMP (cGMP),
(8) SH-containing compounds such as glutathione.

6.3 WHAT DOES VITAMIN C DO?

Prevention and cure of scurvy

There is a consensus of opinion in the scientific world that scurvy is a vitamin C-specific disease, and that death is the end result of vitamin C deprivation. The first accurate documentation of the signs and symptoms of scurvy was provided by Lind in 1757. He demonstrated that oranges and lemons were more effective and rapid than cider in curing the scorbutic patient. However, not everybody took his work seriously, and many people died of scurvy during the following two centuries. At long last in 1928 the antiscorbutic vitamin was isolated from foods and animal tissues; crystalline ascorbic acid was obtained soon afterwards by laboratory and factory synthesis, and methods for its analysis were developed. In 1937 Wolbach redemonstrated that the lack of vitamin C in the human diet is the main cause of:

(1) haemorrhages which may occur anywhere in the body,
(2) profound changes in the structure of the teeth and gums,
(3) changes, deformities and falling apart of bones due to loss of supporting cartilage,
(4) enlargement of heart and damage of heart muscles,
(5) degeneration of muscle fibres,
(6) anaemia due to destruction of blood-forming cells in the bone marrow and loss of blood through haemorrhages,
(7) loss of calcium through degeneration of the bone matrix,
(8) degeneration of the sex organs,
(9) increased metabolic rate or increased oxygen consumption (Sherman, 1946).

These signs and symptoms affect the skin, the mouth, the eyes, the blood, the teeth, the heart, the muscles, the bones and the reproductive system. The metabolism on the whole is disturbed since vitamin C is present in tissues of high metabolic activity and since the vitamin takes part in so many biochemical reactions which are essential for the proper workings of the body.

It is generally accepted that ocular lesions which are considered the most severe symptoms of scurvy develop after about 90 days of complete deprivation of vitamin C. This was found in experimental studies using human volunteers, in whom scurvy was induced (see citations in Irwin and Hutchins, 1976). Two of these studies must be mentioned because they had worldwide repercussions. They were considered by many as providing indisputable evidence that 10 mg of vitamin C, or even less, can cure and prevent scurvy. Meticulously executed, very expensive in terms of person-power and money, one was conducted in Sheffield, England (Bartley, Krebs, and O'Brien, 1953), the other in Iowa City in the United States (Baker *et al.*, 1969; Hodges *et al.*, 1969).

The Sheffield study

This study used volunteers aged 21 to 34 years (19 male and one female), who led a normal life and had no strenuous work. After 6 weeks on a diet providing 70 mg of vitamin C per day, all volunteers were placed on a basal diet containing only 1 mg vitamin C. They were divided into three groups and studied between October 1944 and February 1946 (16 months). All three groups received the basal diet. The control group of three subjects received in addition 70 mg ascorbic acid per day from tablets, and seven subjects were given a 'prophylactic' dose of 10 mg ascorbic acid per day from tablets. The test group of ten subjects (nine males and the one female) received no supplement; three of the men were withdrawn from the experiment because they had serious health problems. Biochemically each individual was tested repeatedly for several parameters and vitamin C was measured in blood plasma, white blood cells, whole blood and urine. The clinical examination was frequent and thorough and the diagnosis of *clinical scurvy* was made when *haemorrhages* in the hair follicles of the forearms and lower limbs appeared. Minor signs such as gingivitis and hyperkeratosis of follicles were not considered as indicative of clinical scurvy.

After 160 days of vitamin C depletion the seven subjects of the test group were given first 10 mg and then 20 mg ascorbic acid from tablets. Three of the seven men in the 10 mg 'prophylactic' group were placed on the basal diet only, for a further 71 days, and then they received 5 mg ascorbic acid from tablets for 125 days. This group did not develop clinical scurvy at any time of the experiment.

The investigators concluded that the *minimum* protective dose of ascorbic acid as measured by the absence of clinical scurvy was ≤ 10 mg. However as measured by physical fatigue, statistical analysis revealed small differences in favour of the group receiving 70 mg ascorbic acid against the group receiving 10 mg. In order to cover 'the requirement of normal adults with their inherent variabilities, enhanced by the variety of their activities and environment' the investigators suggested trebling the minimum protective dose of 10 mg, that is 30 mg for the requirement of the normal adult male and female. They added, however, that this assessment, though having a firmer basis than previous estimates, must be regarded as provisional.

Comments It is interesting to note that the length of time required by doses of 10 mg and 20 mg ascorbic acid to cure clinical scurvy (haemorrhages) ranged from 1 to 18 weeks. On the other hand, administration of much larger amounts of ascorbic acid (3–6 g) to the three subjects who had had serious health problems during the depletion period, improved their conditions, including that of the skin, within a few hours. Two of these men had developed cardiac complications and the third had spinal tuberculosis and had experienced an attack of malaria in the past. This man showed signs of scurvy earlier than the other seven volunteers. On account of these three cases the investigators reported that the original scheme of dosing had to be modified because 'even early stages of vitamin C deficiency might be more dangerous to life than thought at start'. It should be noted further that, although none of the subjects on 10 mg developed clinical scurvy (haemorrhages) in the test period, all had some signs and symptoms usually related to scurvy such as gingivitis, mild hyperkeratosis and slight follicular skin changes. Some of these signs were present also in the three control subjects on 70 mg ascorbic acid per day.

Biochemically the control group maintained blood vitamin C levels around an acceptable range but the group on the 'prophylactic' dose of 10 mg ascorbic acid per day did not. In fact in this group, vitamin C levels in plasma, leukocytes and whole blood fell at the same rate as in the depleted group, and remained around zero in the plasma even during the repletion with either 10 mg or 20 mg ascorbic acid. The authors concluded that such low blood levels are not necessarily detrimental to health since they are not distinguishable from those found in clinical scurvy.

The Iowa study

Baker and his groups studied in 1969 the development of scurvy in six male volunteer prisoners in the state of Iowa, USA and their experiment is known as the Iowa study. It is described in two articles, one by Hodges, Baker *et al.* (1969) and the other by Baker, Hodges *et al.* (1969) in the same journal. They placed prisoners B, Y, L, N, K, and S for 99 days on a vitamin C-free, liquid diet, balanced with other nutrients, and administered by means of a gastric tube. The prisoners were housed in the metabolic ward but were compelled to walk for 10 miles a day and to wear a pedometer at all times. Prisoners B and Y escaped on day 54, so they were left with four prisoners. On day 100 they gave to each prisoner ^{14}C-labelled ascorbic acid in the following dosages:

prisoner L	4 mg
prisoner N	8 mg
prisoner K	16 mg
prisoner S	32 mg

On day 114 the liquid diet was replaced by a solid one which provided an additional 2.5 mg of vitamin C. From day 156 onwards prisoner N received the solid diet (2.5 mg of vitamin C) plus 64 mg of unlabelled ascorbic acid. From day 154 onwards prisoner S was given the 32 mg of ascorbic acid in unlabelled form. The study was ended on day 210, but between days 197 and 210 all subjects received a 500 mg ascorbic acid supplement and an *ad libitum* diet containing about 100 mg vitamin C.

The signs and symptoms of scurvy which were examined were:

(1) hyperkeratosis (thickening of the outer horny layer of the skin),
(2) congestion of follicles (abnormal accumulation of blood in pouch-like depressions of the skin),
(3) petechiae (round red spots) and other skin haemorrhages,
(4) conjunctival lesions (lesions of the membrane lining the eyelids and covering the eyeball),
(5) sublingual haemorrhages,
(6) gum swelling or congestion or both,
(7) bleeding gums,
(8) papillary (papilla = small nipple-like elevation) swelling.

Clinical scurvy was diagnosed when conjunctival lesions developed.

Comments We believe that this experiment indicated that during the depletion period there was *individual variation* between the four prisoners with respect to the development and time of appearance of scurvy symptoms: some had a few symptoms, others had none, some had mild and others severe symptoms. Within 10 days of strict deprivation of vitamin C, hyperkeratosis was present in three of the four prisoners, three had gum swelling or gum congestion or both, one had bleeding gums and two had papillary swelling. After 90 days of depletion all four prisoners had hyperkeratosis but only three had developed conjunctival lesions or clinical scurvy. Equally there was individual variation in the time of disappearance of the symptoms, irrespective of the intake of ascorbic acid of the four prisoners. It is difficult to accept that a dose of 6.5 mg ascorbic acid was sufficient to prevent and cure all symptoms of scurvy in prisoner L. He appeared to be cured in 10 days of some minor sublingual haemorrhages, but he still had hyperkeratosis, conjunctival lesions and gum swelling at the end of the trial. Moreover, the dose of 6.5 mg ascorbic acid per day did not prevent him from developing congestion of follicles, petechial haemorrhages and papillary swelling in between the repletion period. Two of the prisoners (L and N) developed mental and emotional changes which developed concurrently with the objective signs of scurvy (Kinsman and Hood, 1971). All four prisoners had fatiguability of the legs, which limited the length of their daily walks, and a mild general malaise. The Iowa investigators concluded that they had confirmed the results of the Sheffield experiment and made the same recommendation: trebling the dose of 10 mg vitamin C to cover variations in vitamin C requirements of the whole population of adults.

It is difficult to accept, from the results of the Sheffield study (six male and one female adult 'healthy' volunteers) and of the Iowa study (four male prisoners), that a daily intake of 30 mg vitamin C could be sufficient to cover individual variations in vitamin C requirements and to provide additional benefits for all healthy adult men and women around the world.

Can prisoners be considered mentally, socially and clinically normal healthy individuals on whom to base results for extrapolation to groups of people who live outside the prison's walls and do not eat food via a gastric tube? Even if the investigators of both groups arrived at the same conclusion, one should not forget that depletion of vitamin C may cause heart problems (Sheffield study) and mental disturbances (Iowa study), the cure of which required much more than 30 mg vitamin C. In our opinion these two experiments indicated that although symptoms of overt scurvy, such as ocular lesions or skin haemorrhages, appeared about 90 days after withdrawal of vitamin C from the diet, other symptoms occurred much earlier and were not minor; in fact some were severe. Thus there is a progressive malfunction of the body along with the progressive decrease of vitamin C intake as illustrated in Figure 7. The result is overt scurvy and finally death.

Cases of scurvy, although rarer than in the past centuries, are still too frequently reported (see, for example Howells, Palmer, and St. John-Brooks, 1954; Kamien *et al.*, 1974). In the period 1975–79 seven reports of scurvy were made in the medical literature. These included two from women who were on self-imposed 'quack' diets, a warning from two reports that there was a high association between scurvy and Crohn's disease, a dentist report of a middle-aged man, and three cases of infantile scurvy.

The question is: is it medically justified to maintain the body in a desaturation state, neglect minor signs and symptoms of scurvy and consider the condition of hypovitaminosis C as clinically normal?

Prevention and cure of hypovitaminosis C

Hypovitaminosis C is a condition in which typical scurvy symptoms are not apparent but which presents very low levels of vitamin C in blood plasma, tissues and urine. It may be produced by a low intake of vitamin C or by other causes (see Chapter 10). What happens to those individuals who consume regularly, for months or even years, a diet with a vitamin C content just sufficient to prevent clinical scurvy but not enough to maintain the vitamin in all the tissues, which normally contain it, in concentrations adequate for it to attend to its metabolic functions? Does the human organism adapt itself to this condition without any serious consequences or would it perform better were all tissues provided with a generous supply of vitamin C? If these questions could be answered in a simple way, the vitamin C topic would not be as controversial as it is and this book would not have been written. Many

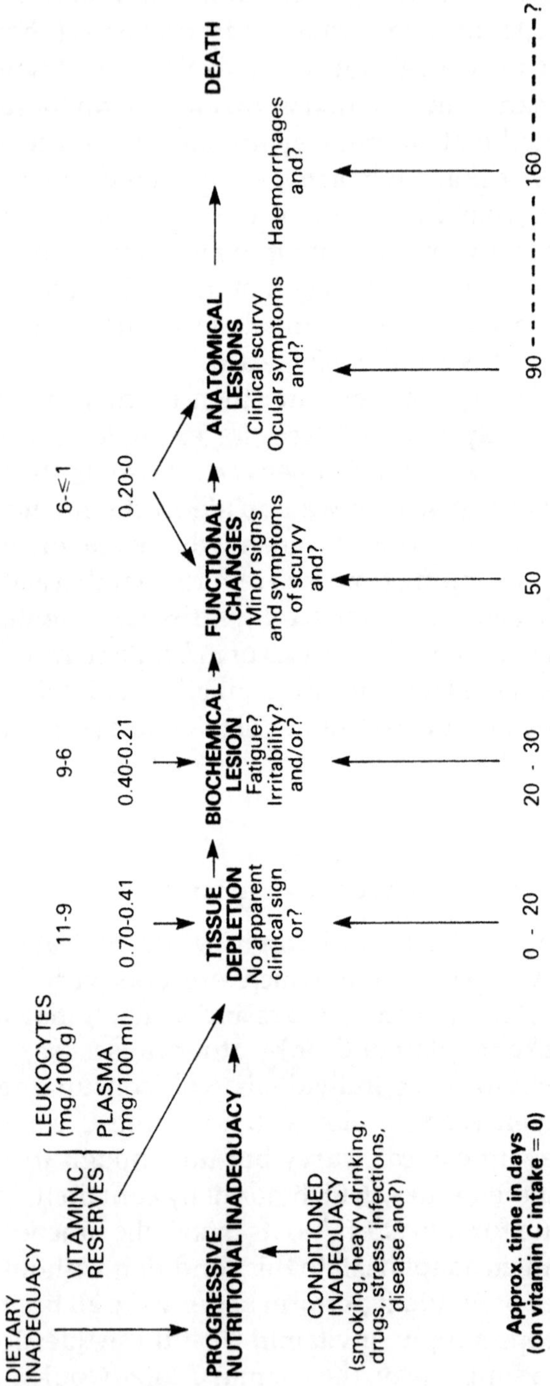

Figure 7 Development of vitamin C deficiency

surveys of the nutritional status of population groups have been carried out in many countries. In every survey it was found, by any standard, that a certain percentage (5, 10, 20% or more) of the population studied had either low intakes of vitamin C and/or low levels of the vitamin in blood plasma, serum, blood cells or urine. The data collected from these surveys are useful but it would be more useful to know what was done about those individuals who were below standards in some nutrient(s), such as vitamin C. They did not have the typical signs and symptoms of scurvy, but were they otherwise healthy and therefore was nothing done for them? Or did they just appear healthy and would have improved their physical and mental performance had they changed their diet to include fresh fruit and vegetables? *Scorbutico* in Italian, the mother tongue of one of the present authors (SN) is an adjective

> 'widely used in a figurative sense to describe an irritable, neurotic, ever-discontented, unsociable, whining, cranky person. The term undoubtedly originated in some of the seaports (Venice, Genoa, Trieste) to which, in earlier times, many seamen must have returned from long journeys suffering from scurvy. Who would not become *'bisbetico, stravagante di carattere e di umore difficile,* i.e. *scorbutico'* when his gums are swollen and bleeding, his legs weak, et cetera?' (Woodhill and Nobile, 1971b).

7
Case studies of scurvy and hypovitaminosis C in Australia

7.1 MENTAL PERFORMANCE OF OLD MEN IN A GERIATRIC HOSPITAL

Out of 49 long-term patients, 11 old men were selected for a vitamin nutrition study in a geriatric hospital in the Sydney area. The plasma levels* of 47 of the 49 men were around 0 mg vitamin C/100 ml. The mean vitamin C intake provided by the hospital diet to the 11 old men was 19 mg/day; it was determined by weighing and analysing each item of food and beverage they consumed during one week – Monday to Sunday (Nobile and Woodhill, 1973). Their plasma levels of vitamin C, which were measured midway in the survey week, ranged from 0.02 to 0.33 mg/100 ml – mean 0.05 mg/100 ml (Woodhill and Nobile, 1972/1973). The 11 men did not have overt scurvy but two of them had perifollicular hyperkeratosis and others had signs of malnutrition. They were a pathetic group with a history of alcoholism and arteriosclerosis, all but one were thin and wasted, and in a poor mental state (Silink, Nobile, and Woodhill, 1972/1973). The exception was not *scorbutico* but alert, cheerful and active. Was this because he supplemented his daily diet with 90 mg ascorbic acid from tablets and had a total vitamin C intake of 113 mg? He was the only one with a plasma level of 0.33 mg vitamin C/100 ml, well above the almost nil levels of the others.

* For classification of plasma levels of vitamin C see Table 11.

A *repletion study* was attempted; five of the 11 men were given 300 mg ascorbic acid per day for 3 days under medical supervision in the hospital. We tested vitamin C daily in their plasma and in 24 hour samples of urine, but no trace of vitamin C could be found at any time. It took administration of 1 g ascorbic acid daily for a further 2–4 days before the plasma vitamin C of all five men reached saturation levels and some vitamin C appeared in the urine (unpublished data).

The *hospital diet was changed* to include better food sources of vitamin C and of other vitamins, because vitamin C was the main but not the only culprit.

A *double-blind study* was made with ten of the men to test their mental performance. Five received a multivitamin–multimineral preparation containing 150 mg ascorbic acid, and five received an identical form of placebo. The mental performance of the men was tested initially and monthly for 3 months by two outside specialists in the field. At the same time the men were clinically examined by the medical consultant in our team and their blood was monitored for vitamin levels. The code was unknown to all persons involved in the study. For various reasons the results could not be published, but they indicated a strong and statistically valid trend towards better mental performance with increasing plasma levels of vitamin C. Mental performance was better in the vitamin group who had the highest plasma levels of vitamin C, but some improvement was noted in those men in the placebo group whose vitamin C levels reflected the change in the hospital diet. There was no evidence of a mental change in those men with persistent low levels of plasma vitamin C, either because they did not eat enough vitamin C or because they were beyond recovery.

7.2 MENTAL PERFORMANCE OF OLD MEN RECEIVING MEALS-ON-WHEELS

For this study we took six old men who received meals-on-wheels 5 days a week and had a mean* vitamin C intake (analysed during 1 week) of 19 mg/day, and a mean† plasma level of 0.076 mg vitamin C/100 ml (Woodhill and Nobile, 1972/1973). They did not have overt scurvy but two men were obese, two had markedly

* Range of intakes: 14 to 30 mg/day
† Range of plasma levels: 0.033 to 0.178 mg/100 ml

wasted subcutaneous tissues, one had a recent history of megaloblastic anaemia precipitated by a respiratory tract infection and a period of very poor eating habits. He had received treatment with folic acid, vitamin B_{12} and iron. At the time of the survey he was not anaemic but his serum and red cell folic acid were both below normal and his vitamin C level in the plasma was around nil (0.08 mg/100 ml) (Silink, Nobile, and Woodhill, 1972/1973). One of these men, though obese, was more active and sociable than the others. He had a grapefruit tree in his garden and occasionally ate the fruit. His intake was just on 30 mg vitamin C/day (the Australian dietary allowance for vitamin C – National Health and Medical Research Council, 1971); his plasma vitamin C level though not high was the highest of the group (0.178 mg/100 ml). The meals-on-wheels provided good sources of calories, protein, carbohydrates and of other vitamins tested (A, B_1, B_2, PP) but vitamin C was in the shortest supply. This is not surprising because the meals were kept hot for about 2 hours in the kitchen and then carried to the men's houses within ½, 1 and 1½ hours. The then Minister of Social Security saw the authors' results and succeeded in introducing a measure to provide each meals-on-wheels service with a 100 ml carton of pure orange juice containing at least 40 mg vitamin C/100 ml or an equivalent source of the vitamin. The two cartons of orange juice tested contained 45 mg vitamin C/100 ml. The results of this government decision could not be monitored, but the distribution of a vitamin C source with meals-on-wheels is still on and hopefully will continue to be practised.

7.3 PRECIPITATION OF SCURVY IN AN OLD WOMAN

The elderly subject was living alone and cooking for herself. She had an intake of 25 mg vitamin C/day (1 week average) and a plasma level of 0.2 mg vitamin C/100 ml. She had 'a long-standing colitis and restricted her intake of fresh fruit and vegetables because they increased her diarrhoea. She had no clinical signs of vitamin C deficiency. Three years later, during an exacerbation of her colitis, she was found to have reddened gums, small sublingual haemorrhages (which are signs and symptoms of scurvy), cheilosis and angular stomatitis.' Her plasma vitamin C was 0.05 mg/100 ml (Silink, Nobile, and Woodhill, 1972/1973).

7.4 ABORIGINAL FAMILIES AND SCURVY BABY

Malnutrition amongst the Aboriginal population is well documented but very little has been done about it. One attempt to improve their diet was made and it helped them; but unfortunately it was discontinued because it hit the press headlines with a sensational and inaccurate report (Kamien *et al.*, 1975a). It is also known that Aboriginal mothers in particular are badly nourished. We measured the nutritional status of two Aboriginal families at Bourke (Western New South Wales) and tested their diet for 6 days (Monday to Saturday). The individual vitamin C intake was analysed; it ranged from 7 to 26 mg/day in one family of ten members and from 7 to 24 mg/day in the other family of seven. The plasma vitamin C levels of the four parents ranged from 0.04 to 0.34 mg/100 ml. They were lower than the plasma vitamin C levels of the children* which ranged from 0.22 to 0.82 mg/100 ml in the eight children of one family and from 0.79 to 1.39 mg/100 ml in the five children of the second family. None of the 17 members of the two families had overt scurvy, but all had either clinical signs of nutritional deficiencies or conditions such as nasal discharge, conjunctivitis, perforated eardrums in the children, and diabetes or infection of the urinary tract in the parents (Kamien *et al.*, 1975b). The mother in one family, who had recurrent urinary tract infection, had a vitamin C intake of 7 mg/day and a plasma level of 0.19 mg/100 ml. She had breastfed a baby girl since birth. At seven months the *baby* developed *clinical scurvy*. Her mother's milk contained only 2 mg vitamin C/100 ml and the only supplementary food the baby received was canned spaghetti which on analysis had nil vitamin C (Kamien *et al.*, 1974).

7.5 ABORIGINAL WOMEN OF CHILDBEARING AGE

We tested vitamin levels in nine Aboriginal women of childbearing age in Bourke on two occasions. They were either non-pregnant, pregnant or breastfeeding at one or the other time of testing. Only one non-pregnant woman had a plasma vitamin C level around 0.7 mg/100 ml. She was 15 years old at that stage but three years later her plasma level was lower (0.4 mg/100 ml). The

* Aboriginal children at Bourke collected empty cans to get some money to buy fruit . . . not lollies!

levels of the other eight women ranged from 0.07 to 0.52 mg vitamin C/100 ml plasma in 1971 and from 0.06 to 0.50 mg vitamin C/100 ml plasma in 1974. Clinically all had some disease conditions; gingivitis was not uncommon nor were dental caries and other clinical signs of malnutrition. Two of the women were prescribed 'megadoses' of folic acid* and iron† but no vitamin C; yet vitamin C is known to act on the metabolism of both folic acid and iron (see Section 6.2). The intake of folic acid was reflected in plasma levels of this vitamin five to ten times higher than 3 ng/ml (normal level) but, on second testing when treatment had ceased the levels had fallen to 0.8 ng/ml and 2.3 ng/ml folic acid respectively. Iron levels in blood were not measured (Kamien *et al.*, 1975a). The Aboriginal mothers studied at Kollarinebri and Walgett in Western New South Wales had similar vitamin C status, as indicated by plasma levels of the vitamin. In this study we found a significant correlation between plasma levels of vitamin C and of folic acid in the women (Nobile, 1974b).

7.6 AUSTRALIAN CHILDREN FROM SOCIOECONOMIC STRESS GROUPS

Children have been found to have higher plasma vitamin C levels than adults on the same intakes (Woodhill, 1979). Nevertheless levels of vitamin C between 0.01 and 0.2 mg/100 ml plasma, which are indicative of hypovitaminosis C, were found in some Australian children from stress groups. We studied six boys aged 3–5 years, whose mothers were widows with large families. Their vitamin C intake with the food ranged, in 1 week, from 8 to 20 mg/day; it was analysed. One of these boys ate only 8 mg of vitamin C/day, had 0.07 mg vitamin C/100 ml plasma and was emotionally disturbed. Another boy was on treatment for gastrointestinal worm infestation. He received 19 mg vitamin C from his food and additionally 25 mg ascorbic acid from a multivitamin syrup; his plasma vitamin C level was 0.2 mg/100 ml. We studied 21 girls in two orphanages. They received a diet which provided from 14 to 36 mg vitamin C/day; there was no difference between the two

* 5 mg folic acid is about 15 times the Australian dietary allowance for this vitamin in pregnancy and lactation.
† 300 mg or 600 mg iron are 20 and 40 times the Australian dietary allowance for iron in pregnancy and lactation (National Health and Medical Research Council, 1971).

orphanages with respect to the preparation and supply of the food. Levels of vitamin C in the range of 0.01–0.2 mg/100 ml plasma were found in two part-Aboriginal girls aged 5 and 6 years who were emotionally disturbed, in one girl who had frequent tonsillitis and in one obese girl aged 11 years with dental caries and mild thyroid enlargement (Woodhill *et al.*, 1974).

7.7 ADULT AUSTRALIANS IN VARYING DEGREES OF HEALTH

We have summarized in Table 5 the number and percentage of 431 adult men and women in varying degrees of health who had plasma vitamin C levels indicative of tissue saturation, marginal status, biochemical deficiency or clinical deficiency – ranging in decreasing order from above 0.7 to 0 mg vitamin C/100 ml plasma. Some of these data are unpublished. The age of the 431 individuals ranged from 18 to 55 years; they were studied between 1969 and 1976. The data reported in Table 5 refer to:

(1) an affluent group of 14 *healthy* subjects who were screened for absence of disease of any type and were not taking any medication or vitamin supplements. Their diet was analysed during 1 week for the content of vitamin C and of other vitamins (Nobile, Woodhill, and Rosevear, 1976). The vitamin C intakes of five subjects ranged from 67 to 130 mg and those of nine subjects from 30 to 60 mg per day;
(2) an affluent group of 55 *apparently healthy* adults who were not examined clinically;
(3) a *socioeconomic stress group* of 24 white Australians and 51 Aborigines;
(4) groups of patients with various *diseases* who had been referred by their doctors for blood vitamin testing including 55 patients with a variety of conditions, 155 patients with specific diseases as listed in Table 5, 77 patients with the diagnosis of *malnutrition* among whom there were 19 patients with symptoms of peripheral neuropathy, malabsorption, deficiency of vitamin A or deficiency of vitamin E (this due to ingestion of large quantities of polyunsaturated fat for a long period), 31 chronic alcoholics with vitamin B_1 deficiency (beri-beri, Wernicke's encephalopathy, Korsa-

Table 5 Number and percentage of adults in varying degrees of health with acceptable, marginal and deficient plasma levels of vitamin C

			Plasma levels of vitamin C									
Group[a]	Description of groups (age 18–55 years)	Number tested	Acceptable tissue saturation		Marginal status		Biochemical deficiency		Clinical deficiency			
			> 0.7 mg		0.41–0.7 mg		0.21–0.4 mg		0.01–0.2 mg		0 mg/100 ml	
			n	(%)	n	(%)	n	(%)	n	(%)	n	(%)
Health												
(1)	'Normals' screened, affluent group, on no medications, on average intakes of vitamin C 67–130 mg/day from food only	5	5	(100)								
(2)	'Normals' screened, affluent group, on no medications on average intakes of vitamin C 30–60 mg/day from food only	9	8	(89)	1	(11)						
Apparent health												
(3)	Apparently healthy, affluent group	55	36	(65)	11	(20)	6	(11)	2	(4)		
(4)	Socioeconomic stress group	24	1	(4)	4	(17)	7	(29)	8	(33)	4	(17)
(5)	Aborigines	51	2	(4)	5	(10)	13	(25)	30	(59)	1	(2)
Disease												
(6)	Patients with a variety of conditions	55	27	(49)	13	(24)	9	(16)	4	(7)	2	(4)
(7)	Patients with specific diseases[b]	155	38	(25)	37	(24)	36	(23)	39	(25)	5	(3)
Malnutrition												
(8)	Patients with symptoms of malnutrition[c]	19	2	(11)	4	(21)			11	(58)	2	(11)
(9)	Alcoholics with symptoms of malnutrition[d]	31					2	(7)	18	(58)	11	(35)
(10)	Patients with various forms of anaemia	18	6	(33)	2	(11)	3	(17)	6	(33)	1	(6)
(11)	Patient with pellagra	1					1	(100)				
(12)	Patients with beri-beri (non-alcoholic)	5							4	(80)	1	(20)
(13)	Patients with scurvy	3							1	(33)	2	(67)
	Total	431	125	(29)	77	(18)	77	(18)	123	(28)	29	(7)

[a] The subjects were not taking vitamin supplements

[b] Including thyroidism $n = 13$; cataract and renal failure $n = 33$; renal failure on maintenance haemodialysis $n = 20$; paraplegia $n = 23$; oral lesions $n = 19$; porphyria $n = 14$; Parkinson's disease $n = 7$, schizophrenia $n = 21$

[c] Including peripheral neuropathy, malabsorption, vitamin A or E deficiency

[d] Including chronic alcoholics and patients with beri-beri, Wernicke's encephalopathy and Korsakoff's syndrome

koff's syndrome), 18 patients with various forms of anaemia, one patient with pellagra, five patients with beri-beri not caused by alcoholism, and three patients with scurvy, one of whom was an alcoholic.

Levels of vitamin C in the plasma ranging from 0 to 0.2 mg/100 ml, classified in Table 5 as indicative of clinical deficiency, are considered low by any standard. They were found in overt scurvy (100%), but were prevalent also in other deficiency diseases such as beri-beri whether due to alcoholism (93%) or not (100%). They were found in general malnutrition (69%), in various forms of anaemia (39%), in patients with specific diseases (28%), or other clinical conditions (11%). These low plasma vitamin C levels were present also in the groups of apparently healthy individuals under socioeconomic stress, whether black (61%) or white (50%) and even in the affluent class of Australian (4%). The figures in brackets indicate the percentage of subjects in each group with levels of vitamin C in the plasma ranging from 0 to 0.2 mg/100 ml. All those individuals were in the condition of *hypovitaminosis* C. The fact that cases of scurvy, beri-beri, pellagra and deficiency of the vitamins A and E were analysed for vitamin levels indicates that vitamin malnutrition existed in Australia at least until 1976.

Table 6 Blood vitamin profile in acute cardiac beri-beri from alcoholism (225 g alcohol/day) (Nobile, 1979) – male 40–50-year-old garbage collector

Time	*Levels of vitamins per 100 ml plasma*				*Functional tests in erythrocytes Coenzyme % reactivation*		
	C mg	A IU	ProA μg	E mg	B_1 TPP %	B_2 FAD %	B_6 PALP %
Day 0	0.02[a]	299[d]	0[a]	0.53[b]	63[a]	0[c]	30[c]
Day 1*	0.04[a]	140[c]	0[a]	0.29[a]	4[c]	6[b]	30[c]
Day 2*	0.04[a]	149[c]	0[a]	0.37[a]	0[c]	0[c]	31[c]

* After injection of 50 mg vitamin B_1
[a] Deficient; [b] marginal; [c] acceptable; [d] above normal
ProA = beta-carotene; TPP = thiamine pyrophosphate; FAD = flavin adenine dinucleotide; PALP = pyridoxal-5′-phosphate

Table 7 Blood vitamin profile in Wernicke's encephalopathy from alcoholism (Nobile,1979) – male 48 years old

Time	*Levels of vitamins per 100 ml plasma*					*Functional tests in erythrocytes Coenzyme % reactivation*		
	C mg	A IU	ProA µg	E mg	B_c ng	B_1 TPP %	B_2 FAD %	B_6 PALP %
Day 0*	0[a]	380[d]	0[a]	0.86[c]	1300[c]	63[a]	30[a]	26[c]
Day 13†	0.08[a]	122[c]	8[a]	0.58[b]	4600[d]	4[c]	–	25[c]

* Diagnosis: mildly confused, with vertical and horizontal nystagmus, a wide base staggering gait and bilateral VI nerve palsies
† Medical comments (for follow-up after appropriate treatment): bilateral VI nerve palsies disappeared within 16 hours after injection of 50 mg B_1 but nystagmus remained
Other treatment: Penicillin 250 mg a.i.d., vitaminorum caps. (vitamin C: 15 mg; PP: 7 mg; B_1: 1 mg; B_2: 0.5 mg; A: 2500 IU; D: 300 IU) t.d.s. B_c: 5 mg t.d.s.
[a] Deficient; [b] marginal; [c] acceptable; [d] above normal
ProA = beta-carotene; B_c = folic acid; TPP = thiamine pyrophosphate; FAD = flavin adenine dinucleotide; PALP = pyridoxal-5'-phosphate

Correlations with dietary intakes and white blood cell concentrations have indicated that plasma levels are good indices of vitamin C status (see Section 9.1) (Sauberlich, Dowdy, and Skala, 1974). In view of the interaction of vitamin C in so many metabolic pathways, and with so many nutrients, it would seem logical to expect that correction of vitamin C deficiency would improve the condition of the malnourished patient and of patients with various diseases. The blood vitamin profile of the alcoholic with acute cardiac beri-beri illustrated in Table 6 shows that this patient had biochemical deficiency not only of vitamin B_1 but also of vitamin C, which was not corrected by the administration of large doses of vitamin B_1 alone. The case of Wernicke's encephalopathy reported in Table 7 was equally deficient in both vitamins. Although he received, besides the usual treatment with 50 mg vitamin B_1, 45 mg ascorbic acid per day from multivitamin tablets, this dose was not sufficient to correct the plasma level of vitamin C which remained around 0 after 13 days. It is recognized that scurvy is a vitamin C-related disease, but in the case shown in Table 8 the

Table 8 Blood vitamin profile in scurvy from alcoholism (Nobile, 1979) – male 32 years old, heavy drinker, eats little fruit

Time	*Levels of vitamins per 100 ml plasma*				*Functional tests in erythrocytes Coenzyme % reactivation*		
	C mg	A IU	ProA μg	E mg	B_1 TPP %	B_2 FAD %	B_6 PALP %
Day 0*	0[a]	76[a]	0[a]	0.49[b]	70[a]	0[c]	106[a]
Day 16†	1.07[c]	164[c]	0[a]	0.57[b]	12[c]	0[c]	47[c]

* Diagnosis: Stiff, swollen and bruised ankles, occasional gum bleeding and gum hypertrophy, chronic liver disease
† After treatment with 100 mg ascorbic acid t.d.s
[a] Deficient; [b] marginal; [c] acceptable
ProA = beta-carotene; TPP = thiamine pyrophosphate; FAD = flavin adenine dinucleotide; PALP = pyridoxal-5′-phosphate

alcoholic had biochemical deficiency of vitamin C and also of vitamins A, B_1, B_6, and of the pro-vitamin A. Administration of 300 mg ascorbic acid/day for 16 days appeared to have produced levels of vitamin C in the plasma indicative of tissue saturation and normalized, at the same time, the levels of the other vitamins (Nobile, 1979). In a study on oral lichen planus it was found that 49% of the 41 patients showed good improvement, and 22% some improvement of the condition, when biochemical deficiency of all the vitamins tested was corrected and vitamin C in the plasma approached tissue saturation levels (Jolly and Nobile, 1977).

8
How much vitamin C do we humans need? – dietary allowances

The need for a yardstick to assess the nutritional adequacy of dietary intakes was recognized at the end of the Second World War. Allowances for calories and nutrients were needed to plan for reconstruction after the food crisis caused by the war. In one or two countries, committees of nutrition experts made recommendations on intakes of essential nutrients which could be recommended for planning food requirements. Vitamin C was one of the nutrients included in the tables of recommendations and, in the postwar period up to the present time, the recommendations for the daily intake of vitamin C for humans have been going up and down like a yo-yo. The questions which the committees of expert nutritionists had to try to answer were:

(1) How much vitamin C do healthy men and women need?
(2) Do mothers-to-be and nursing mothers, growing children and the elderly need more or less vitamin C than adult healthy men and women?

The nutritional scientists have not been able to answer these questions due to a lack of knowledge about the biochemical and physiological functions of vitamin C. Functional tests for assessing vitamin status are available for some other vitamins, but not for vitamin C. No such tests have been worked out for vitamin C because neither its precise metabolic function, nor how many enzyme systems need it, nor how many hormones are dependent on it are known.

In the early years following the discovery of vitamin C, the nutritional scientists (Todhunter and Robbins, 1940; Sherman, 1946) accepted that:

(1) the absence of scurvy does not prove that the food is supplying as much vitamin C as the body needs for 'its best health, vigour and ability to resist disease';
(2) plasma levels of vitamin C were good indices of vitamin C status and reflected intakes of the vitamin, for example, 60 mg intake → 1.00–1.17 mg vitamin C/100 ml plasma; 120 mg intake → about 1.4 mg vitamin C/100 ml plasma;
(3) tissue saturation, that is, 'the condition in which the body shows little disposition to add further to its concentration of vitamin C', was reflected in levels of 1.4–1.7 mg vitamin C/100 ml plasma and only when such levels were reached did urinary excretion of vitamin C increase substantially (Todhunter and Robbins, 1940);
(4) there is individual variation 'in the amount of vitamin C contained in the body, in the rate at which it is destroyed and in the rate at which it leaves the body through the kidneys' (Sherman, 1946).

8.1 SCURVY PREVENTION VERSUS TISSUE SATURATION: THE GREAT DEBATE

The great debate in the committees has been whether scurvy prevention or tissue saturation should be used as a baseline for estimating dietary allowances. In 1946 Sherman reported that there was already then, some difference of opinion as to the benefits of keeping the body saturated with vitamin C, because people had been known to live for relatively long periods, if not indefinitely, at lower intakes of vitamin C without developing specific symptoms of scurvy. But the scientists who had studied vitamin C favoured the concept of tissue saturation because they recognized that before the symptoms of scurvy appear a period of poor health may occur and may sometimes become chronic. This manifests itself in loss of energy, fleeting pains in joints and limbs in adults, and irritability and retarded growth in children: symptoms which disappear when the vitamin C intake is increased. These early scientists accepted the evidence from several human experiments showing that best results (in human performance) were to be expected when the vitamin C content of food and the resulting concentration in the body were kept not only above, but *far* above scurvy levels. The evidence came from the following experiments:

(1) studies of intake levels in animals and man relative to the maintenance of specific functions, such as wound healing, enzyme activity, cellular proliferation and resistance to physiological stress;
(2) tests of tissue storages at different levels of intakes with related observations of tissue injury or functional impairment;
(3) studies of the amount of vitamin C supplied to infants by human milk (containing about 4 mg vitamin C/100 g) which indicated that in these infants plasma levels and urinary excretion of the vitamin approximated the range found in the saturated state of children and adults;
(4) comparative studies in nutrition including animals that require vitamin C (guinea pigs and primates) and animals that maintain a normal concentration of vitamin C by tissue synthesis: in the animals, which can make their own vitamin C, the concentrations in all tissues were higher than in human subjects on ordinary or conventional diets. To meet the levels of vitamin C of these animals, man would have to consume at least 60 mg vitamin C daily (Todhunter and Robbins, 1940; Sherman, 1946; National Research Council/Food and Nutrition Board (United States), 1948).

The evidence, provided by these early research workers who had studied vitamin C, was accepted by the Food and Nutrition Board (FNB) of the National Research Council (NRC) of the United States, who set the dietary allowances for Americans in 1941, 1944, 1948 and 1958 (see Figure 8 for the 'reference' healthy adult man and woman).

The evidence was not acceptable to the nutrition experts of the United Kingdom, Canada, Norway, the Food and Agricultural Organizations (FAO), the World Health Organization (WHO) and Australia (from 1965 onwards). These countries based their recom-

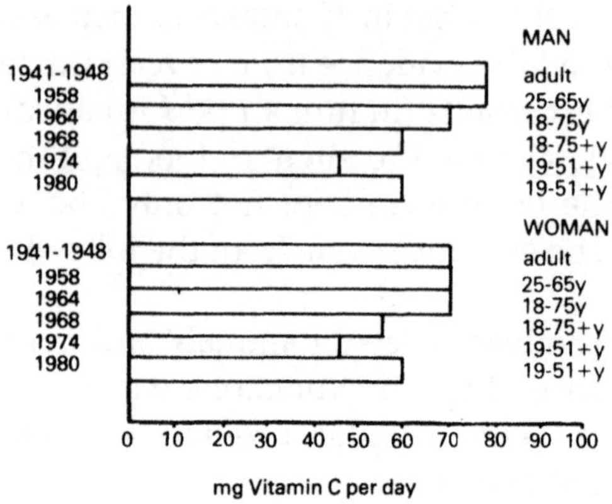

Figure 8 Comparison of dietary allowances for vitamin C recommended in the United States from 1941 to 1980 for the 'reference' healthy adult man and woman

mendations on those made by the investigators of the Sheffield and Iowa studies (see Figure 9).

8.2 DIETARY ALLOWANCES FOR VITAMIN C BASED ON SCURVY PREVENTION

Dietary allowances in the United Kingdom

The British Medical Association in 1950 had recommended an intake of 20 mg vitamin C per day. Following the results of the Sheffield trial (Bartley, Krebs and O'Brien, 1953) the Department of Health and Social Security of the United Kingdom (1969) increased the allowance to 30 mg vitamin C per day to include a 'reasonable margin of safety for adults'. The latest (Department of Health and Social Security, 1979) recommended dietary allowance is still 30 mg vitamin C per day for males and females aged 15–75+ years, 60 mg for pregnancy and lactation, 25 mg for boys and girls aged 9–14 years, and 20 mg for children of other age groups including infants for whom the allowance in 1969 was 15 mg. The reasoning is: 'in the UK few of us are saturated with the vitamin (C), but we do not appear to suffer any ill effects as a result'. Therefore they support the view 'that recommended intakes should be based on an amount sufficient to prevent signs of deficiency'. They state that 'available data provide no reason to alter the allowance for different sexes, for differences in physical activity, or for increasing age'. They accept that requirements are increased during periods of stress (at least in animals) and to achieve satisfactory wound-healing. Although little is known about individual variations, they accept that this may be large (Department of Health and Social Security, 1969; 1979).

Dietary allowances of United Nations agencies FAO/WHO

In 1970 FAO/WHO set their first dietary allowances for 'ascorbic acid (vitamin C)'. They recognized that ascorbic acid has a role in wound-healing but stated that the evidence on its effects on infection, stress and detoxication is equivocal. They based their recommendations on:

(1) the scorbutic prisoner of the Iowa study (Baker *et al.*, 1969; Hodges *et al.*, 1969) in whom 6.5 mg vitamin C were said to cure (?) scurvy;
(2) the findings by Baker (1967) that well-fed men on 75–350 mg vitamin C per day metabolized only 21.5 mg ± 8.1 of the vitamin; and
(3) the survey of 29 countries (mostly underdeveloped) conducted from 1957 to 1971 by the United States Interdepartmental Committee on Nutrition for National Defense (ICNND). This survey had shown that:

(a) scurvy was no longer a public health problem but still occurred sporadically.
(b) low plasma levels of vitamin C indicating inadequate intake were often encountered.
(c) most well-nourished persons had plasma levels above 0.3 mg vitamin C/100 ml;
(d) because plasma levels equal to or above 0.2 mg vitamin C/100 ml were found in large numbers of people with no evidence of deficiency, they considered a level of 0.2 mg/100 ml as acceptable, although plasma levels do not necessarily indicate a true deficiency.
(e) comparison of man with other animals is not valid because the animals who can make their own vitamin C maintain levels in the plasma above 0.4 mg/100 ml, a value con-

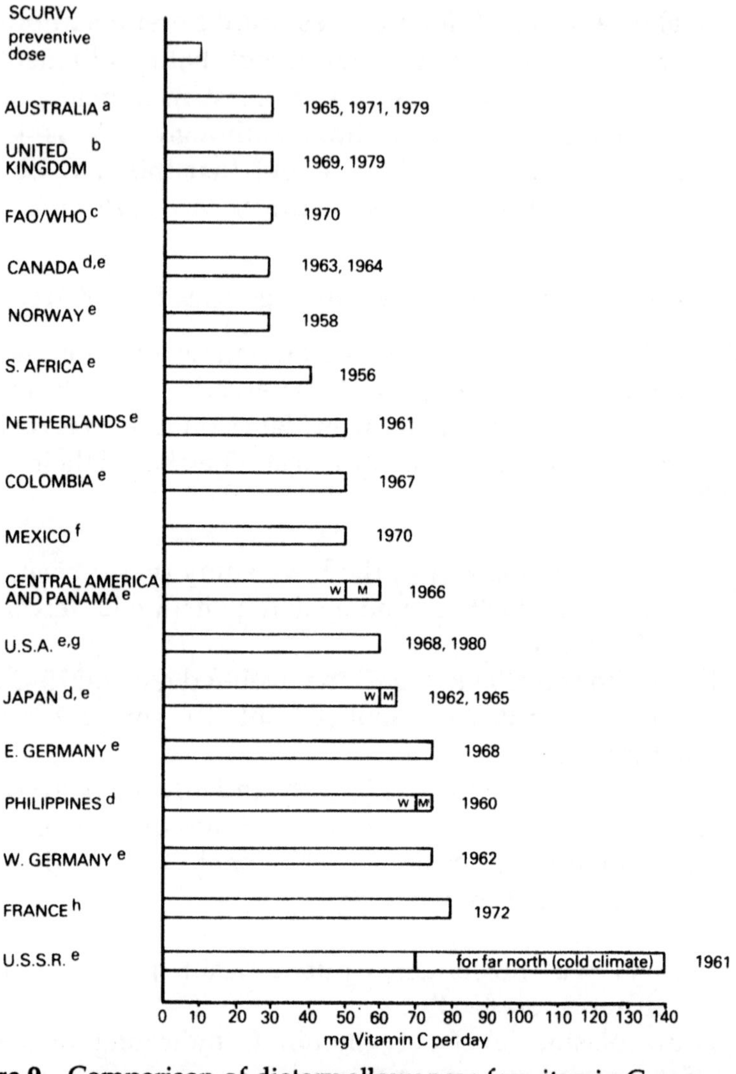

Figure 9 Comparison of dietary allowances for vitamin C recommended in 16 countries and 2 United Nations agencies from 1956 to 1980 for the 'reference' healthy adult man and woman

[a] National Health and Medical Research Council (NH and MRC), (1965). Dietary Allowances for Australians, Canberra; (1971). Dietary Allowances for Use in Australia, Canberra; (1979). Dietary Allowances for Use in Australia, Canberra.

[b] Department of Health and Social security, (1969) Recommended Intakes of Nutrients for the United Kingdom, Reports on Public Health and Medical Subjects No. 120, (1979) Recommended Daily Amounts of Food Energy and Nutrients for Groups of People in the United Kingdom. Reports on Health and Social Subjects 15, (London: HMSO).

[c] Food and Agriculture Organisation of the United Nations (FAO/WHO) (1970) Requirements of Ascorbic Acid, Vitamin D, Vitamin B_{12}, Folate, and Iron, Report of a Joint FAO/WHO Expert Group, Rome.

sidered high by the ICNND – Interdepartmental Committee on Nutrition for National Defense – (1963).

The FAO/WHO group of nutrition experts concluded that 30 mg/day ascorbic acid should be sufficient to prevent scurvy in the adult.

8.3 DIETARY ALLOWANCES FOR VITAMIN C BASED ON THE CONCEPT OF APPROACHING TISSUE SATURATION

Dietary allowances in the United States

The National Research Council (NRC), Food and Nutrition Board (FNB) of the United States stated in 1948 that they had based their recommendations on a conservative appraisal of all evidence available (see Section 8.1). They stated further that the recommended dietary allowances are to be considered

> not as saturation levels, but levels of intake high enough above minimal requirements to cover substantially all individual variations in requirement of normal people and permit additional benefit, and that the evidence from many research laboratories had shown that the intakes of vitamin C recommended were adequate to protect against the classical and the less severe signs and symptoms of scurvy, all individuals: infants to full maturity.

It is interesting to note that the amounts of vitamin C in milligrams (mg) recommended by the NRC/FNB of the United States for every age and sex group were, until 1958, almost the same as

---

[d] National Research Council, Food and Nutrition Board (NRC/FNB) (1964) Recommended Dietary Allowances, Sixth revised edition, National Academy of Sciences, Publication 1146, Washington, DC, p. 58.

[e] National Research Council, Food and Nutrition Board (NRC/FNB) (1968) Recommended Dietary Allowances, Seventh edition, National Academy of Sciences, Publication 1694, Washington, DC, p. 68.

[f] Bourges, H., Chavez, A. and Arroyo P. (1970). Recommendaciones de Nutrimentos para la Poblacion Mexicana, Publicacion L 17 de la Division de Nutricion, Instituto Nacional de Nutricion, Mexico.

[g] National Research Council, Food and Nutrition Board (NRC/FNB) (1980) Recommended Dietary Allowances, Ninth revised edition, National Academy of Sciences, Washington, DC.

[h] Randoin, L., Le Gallic, P., Dupuis, Y. and Bernardin, A. (1972). Tables des Composition des Aliments, Institut Scientifique d'Hygiene Alimentaire, Jacques Lanore Editeur, Paris.

the recommended amounts of protein in grams (Sherman, 1946). Protein is related to kilograms of body weight.

8.4 THE YO–YO OF DIETARY ALLOWANCES FOR VITAMIN C

The differences of opinion between the nutrition committees of various countries and United Nations agencies as to the level of vitamin C needed daily by the 'reference' healthy man and woman are evident from Figure 9. Australia, the United Kingdom, FAO/ WHO, Canada and Norway selected an allowance said to be sufficient to prevent overt signs of scurvy (30 mg); South Africa was a bit more generous (40 mg); and more generous still were the Netherlands, Colombia and Mexico (50 mg). Central America and Panama recommended a still higher allowance for men (60 mg) but allowed less (55 mg) for woman. The United States now allows

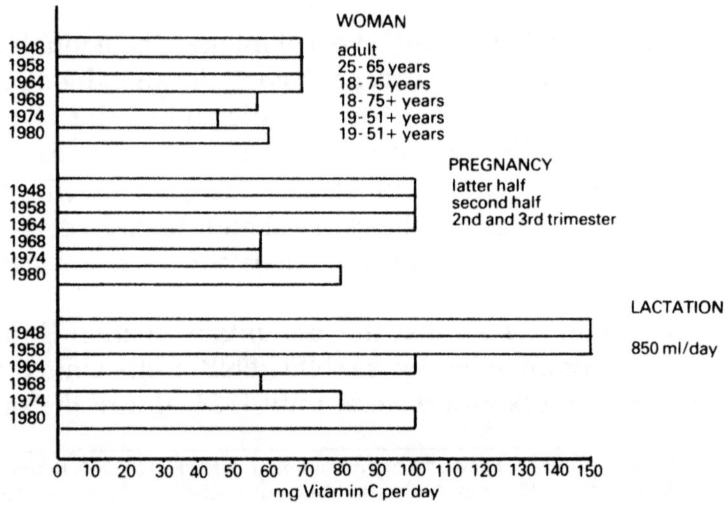

Figure 10 Comparison of dietary allowances for vitamin C recommended in the United States from 1948 to 1980 for women, and in pregnancy and lactation

60 mg for men and women. Japan recommended 60 mg for women and 65 mg for men; East Germany 70 mg for both sexes; the Philippines 70 mg for women and 75 mg for men; West

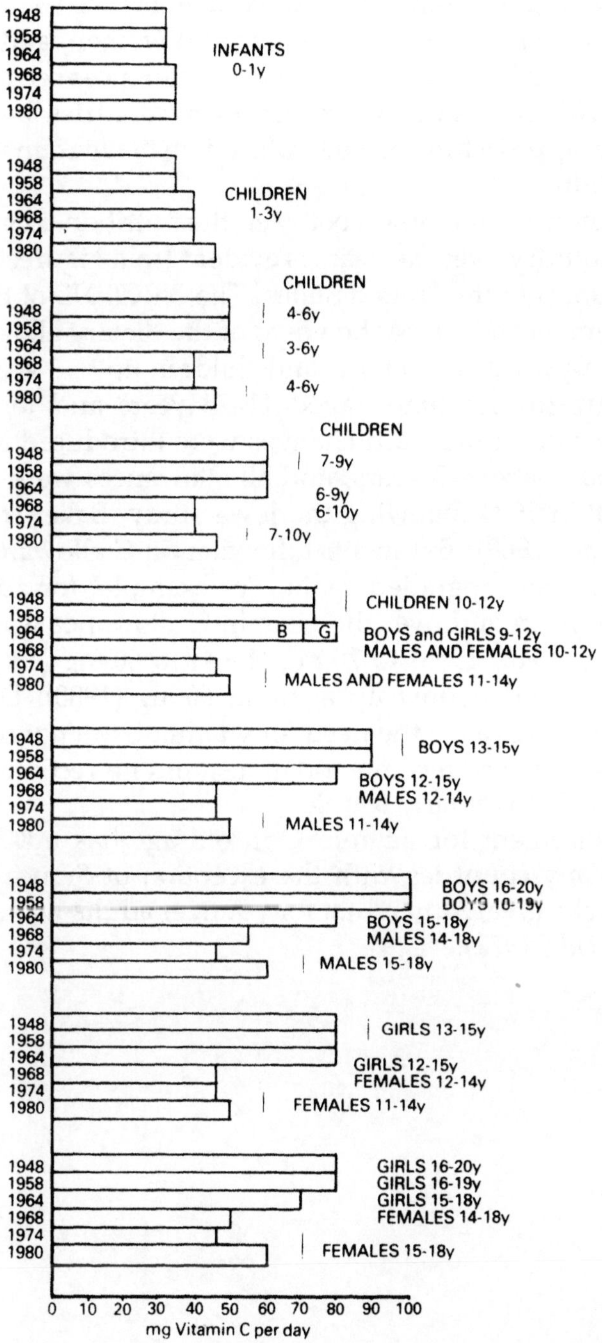

Figure 11 Comparison of dietary allowances for vitamin C recommended in the United States from 1948 to 1980 for infants and children

Germany 75 mg for both men and women; France 80 mg for both sexes; and Russia 70 mg for both men and women, and 140 mg if they live far north in colder climates (for references see footnote to Figure 9). This shows that these last seven countries favoured the concept of approaching tissue saturation of vitamin C for the healthy adults.

The differences of opinion between the nutrition committees of the same country over the years is evident from Figures 8, 10, and 11 with respect to the United States. The NRC/FNB of the United States commenced in 1964 the yo-yo of the dietary allowances for vitamin C: upwards for infants and children up to 3 years of age, and downwards for males aged 11–75 years and for lactating women. Further downward changes were introduced in 1968 for all age groups above 3 years, and all allowances were cut down further still in 1974 following the Iowa study (Baker *et al.*, 1969; Hodges *et al.*, 1969). But in 1980 the vitamin C allowances for all age groups were upgraded again. For example, for adult males aged 19–51 years and over the vitamin C allowance was reduced from 75 mg (1948, 1958) to 70 mg (1964) to 60 mg (1968) and to 45 mg (1974) and is now up again at 60 mg (1980). Differences between the sexes as to the need for vitamin C are not considered in the 1974 and 1980 recommendations, and no recommendation was ever made for elderly people.

The requirement for vitamin C in old age has not been considered in any countries with the exception of France where in 1972 an intake greater than that for younger adults was suggested (Randoin *et al.*, 1972).

9
Assessment of vitamin C status

9.1 CLINICAL, DIETARY AND BIOCHEMICAL ASSESSMENT

All three aspects of vitamin C status – clinical, dietary and biochemical – are important and each one reinforces the other. The clinical evaluation gives a judgement of the nutritional and other related health problems which have been followed by the subject to date. The dietary assessment can give the current status and a long-term estimation of intake. The biochemical assessment can measure what is the status in the body at the time of sampling.

Clinical assessment

The World Health Organization (1963) has suggested a list of signs which can be used in clinical nutrition evaluation. As shown in Table 9, the areas which should be examined are: hair, face, eyes, lips, tongue, gums, glands, skin, nails, subcutaneous tissues, muscular and skeletal systems, gastrointestinal, nervous and cardiovascular systems. Vitamin C should not be assessed in isolation from other nutrients and from the general lifestyle of the subject. Consumption of drugs, alcohol and cigarettes should be considered. A medical history and a routine physical examination is performed, with particular note made of symptoms relating to possible malabsorption. The following anthropometric measurements are noted: height, weight, skinfolds, limb and trunk

Table 9 Clinical assessment of vitamin C status (World Health Organization, 1963)

Area of examination	*Clinical signs*	*Area of examination*	*Clinical signs*
Hair	lack of lustre	*Nails*	koilonychia
	easy pluckability	*Subcutaneous*	skinfold measurement
Face	nasolabial seborrhoea		– midtriceps in female;
Eyes	nightblindness		subscapular in male;
	xerophthalmia (including		oedema
	keratomalacia)	*Muscular and*	haematomas
	Bitot's spots (?)	*skeletal systems*	kyphoscoliosis
	angular palpebritis		fractures
	circum corneal injection		myotatic irritability
	corneal vascularization		muscle tenderness
Lips	angular stomatitis	*Gastrointesinal*	hepatomegaly
	angular scars		ascites
	cheilosis	*Nervous system*	personality change
	rhagades		psychomotor disturbance
Tongue	geographical tongue		mental confusion
	scarlet and raw tongue		sensory loss
	magenta tongue		motor weakness
	atrophic papillae, fissured		loss of position sense
	tongue		loss of vibration sense
Gums	spongy bleeding gums		loss of ankle and knee jerks
Glands	thyroid enlargement		calf tenderness
Skin	xerosis	*Cardiovascular*	cardiac failure
	perifollicular congestion	*system*	peripheral vascular
	follicular hyperkeratosis		dysfunction
	types I and II		
	curled or broken hairs		
	petechiae		
	ecchymoses		
	pellagrous dermatitis		
	Hess test		

measurements. The mental state, adequacy of teeth and dentures, the presence of gastrointestinal, endocrine or metabolic disorders are recorded. The appetite or lack of it at any time, periods of high consumption of empty calorie foods, or of excessive intake of alcohol, cigarettes and medications of any type are all of interest in the assessment of vitamin C status.

Dietary assessment

It is impossible to expect an accurate record of food intake because all methods of dietary assessment as listed in Table 10 have some limitations (Woodhill, 1979). However, an attempt should be made to determine the current intake of food and the amount of vitamin C it provides and to estimate the long-term dietary history of the subject. The consumption of vitamin tablets and the percent-

Table 10 Methods of dietary assessment (Woodhill, 1979)

Method	*Pro*	*Con*
Metabolic ward balance studies weighed and analysed input and output	measures the *status quo*	expensive; no data on food habits
*7-Consecutive day weighed and analysed intakes	accurate intakes (week-days and weekends)	expensive; no data on long-term food habits
3-Day weighed intakes	accurate intakes	as above plus weekend problem
7-Day food logs	staff cost savings	less accurate intakes; no data on long-term food habits
1-Day weighed intakes or food log	spot check	need to repeat test many times to assess food habits
**Dietary history interview	cost savings; estimate of long-term food habits	less accurate intakes
Combination of * and **	estimate of long-term food habits; accurate intakes	expensive

age of total calories coming from sugar, empty calorie foods and alcohol must be included in the dietary history. The intake of vitamin C should be correlated with the clinical and biochemical findings. The recommended dietary allowance of the country is considered as a yardstick for assessing the adequacy of intake of a nutrient. With respect to vitamin C (see Figure 9), adequacy of the intake will depend upon the recommendations of the country in question. An intake of 30 mg vitamin C/day would be considered adequate in the United Kingdom but would be too low in the United States which recommends an intake of 60 mg/day vitamin C.

Biochemical assessment

This measures the state of the body when the samples are taken. Both blood and urine should be examined for all vitamins and iron because of the interrelationships of vitamin C with other vitamins and its effect on iron absorption. Measurement of vitamin C levels in the blood plasma indicates the amount of vitamin C available for transport from one tissue to the other, wherever needed, or to the kidneys for excretion in the urine. The white blood cells or leukocytes store high levels of vitamin C when the body tissues are fully saturated. The main function of the leukocytes is to protect the body from infections by a process called phagocytosis. Measurement of vitamin C levels in these blood cells will provide information on the vitamin C reserves of the body. The amount of vitamin C which was not utilized by the body will be found in the urine as intact ascorbic acid while the amount used up in the metabolic processes will be indicated by the levels of the end-products of vitamin C catabolism (see Section 6.1). As a result of our studies we have classified plasma levels of vitamin C, as indicated in Table 11. The plasma vitamin C levels considered indicative of tissue saturation are those found in a group of adult men and women from the affluent class, who were screened for health by medical examination and were not on medications nor on vitamin supplements. Their dietary intakes of vitamin C (67–130 mg) appeared to be sufficient to ensure tissue saturation levels in the blood plasma comparable to those of a similar group of subjects who were taking 1 g/day ascorbic acid from tablets. Plasma levels classified as 'clinical deficiency' (in other words, in the range from 0 to 0.2 mg vitamin C/100 ml plasma) are those found in overt scurvy and other malnutrition diseases. Although such low levels may not be indicative of clinical scurvy (Bartley, Krebs, and O'Brien, 1953), they certainly show that very little or no vitamin C is available for transport to the tissues which would need it for metabolic functions. The ranges of plasma vitamin C concentrations considered to be marginal or indicative of biochemical deficiency are tentatively classified in Table 11. To obtain information on the vitamin C status both at the time of sampling and on a long-term basis, vitamin C should be measured in the plasma and in the leukocytes and the results should be correlated with the clinical and dietary findings.

9.2 CORRELATIONS BETWEEN CLINICAL, DIETARY AND BIOCHEMICAL VITAMIN C STATUS IN ADULTS

The development of vitamin C deficiency, leading to scurvy and

Table 11 Classification of blood plasma levels of vitamin C (Nobile, 1979)

Interpretation	*mg Vitamin C/100 ml plasma range of values*
Tissue saturation (acceptable)	0.71–1.5
Marginal status	0.41–0.7
Biochemical deficiency	0.21–0.4
Clinical deficiency	0–0.2

death, with progressive nutritional inadequacy was illustrated in Figure 7 (page 74), showing the time relationship with vitamin C levels in plasma and leukocytes and progressive clinical deterioration. A statistically significant correlation between clinical, dietary and biochemical status of vitamin C was found by Bermond and Rilliet (1975). In Figure 12 we show the correlation between plasma, white blood cells, whole blood and intake of vitamin C, as adapted from Bartley, Krebs, and O'Brien (1953). It indicates that doses of vitamin C certainly well above 20 mg/day (around 70 mg) are necessary to maintain levels in the plasma and leukocytes approaching tissue saturation. It also shows that excess vitamin C (600 mg) is stored in the white blood cells.

9.3 SEX AND AGE DIFFERENCE – INTAKE AND PLASMA LEVELS OF VITAMIN C

Figure 13 shows a difference between the sexes and ages. On the same intake, girls had slightly higher plasma levels than boys (not significant) and all children had higher plasma levels than adults and elderly people. The sex difference is apparent in adult men and women and reached significant levels in the elderly (Woodhill, 1979). Similar findings relative to sex and age difference were reported by Dodds (1969), and by Wilson's group (Loh and Wilson, 1971c; Wilson, 1974). These differences should be considered in the assessment of vitamin C status.

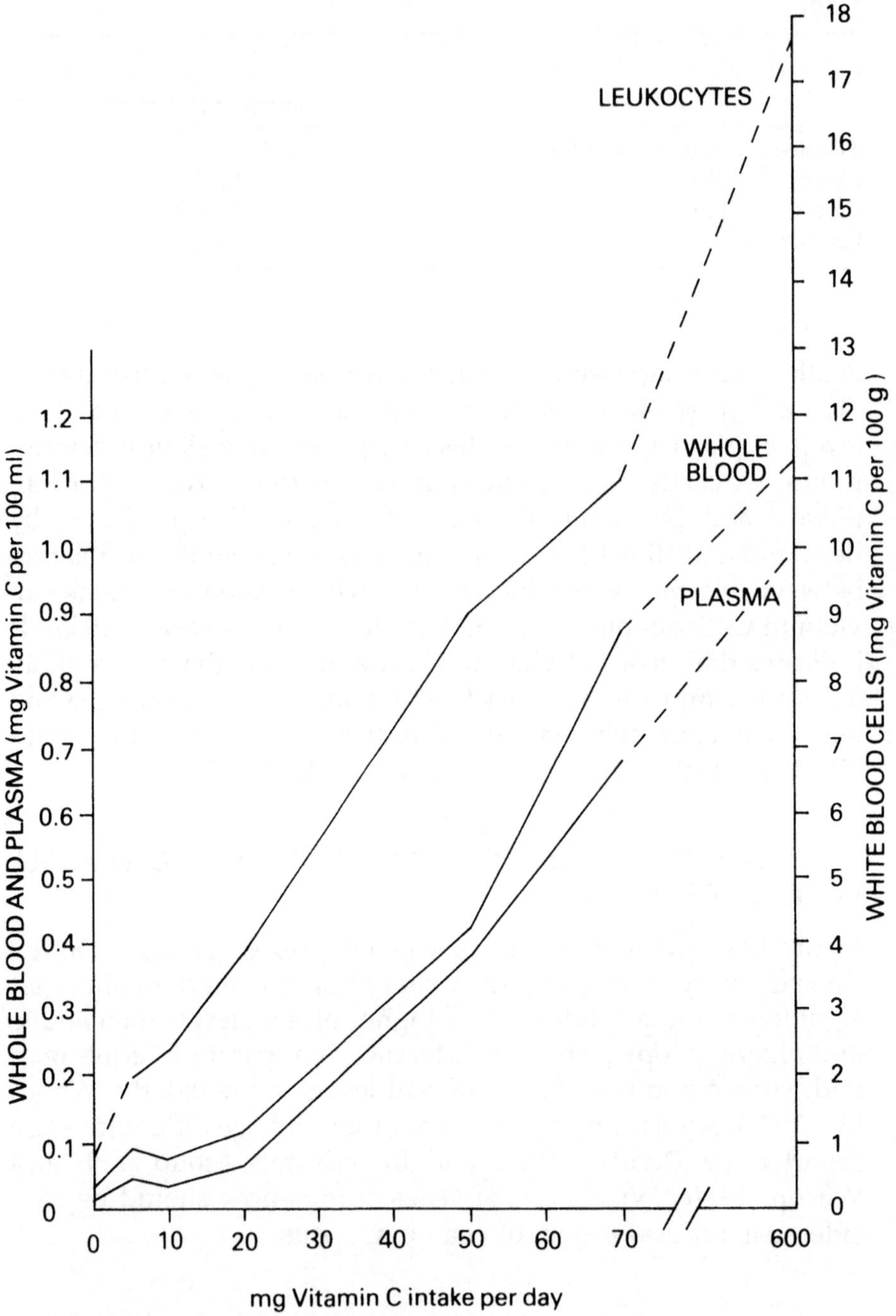

Figure 12 Correlation between dietary and biochemical vitamin C status in adults (adapted from Bartley, Krebs, and O'Brien, 1953)

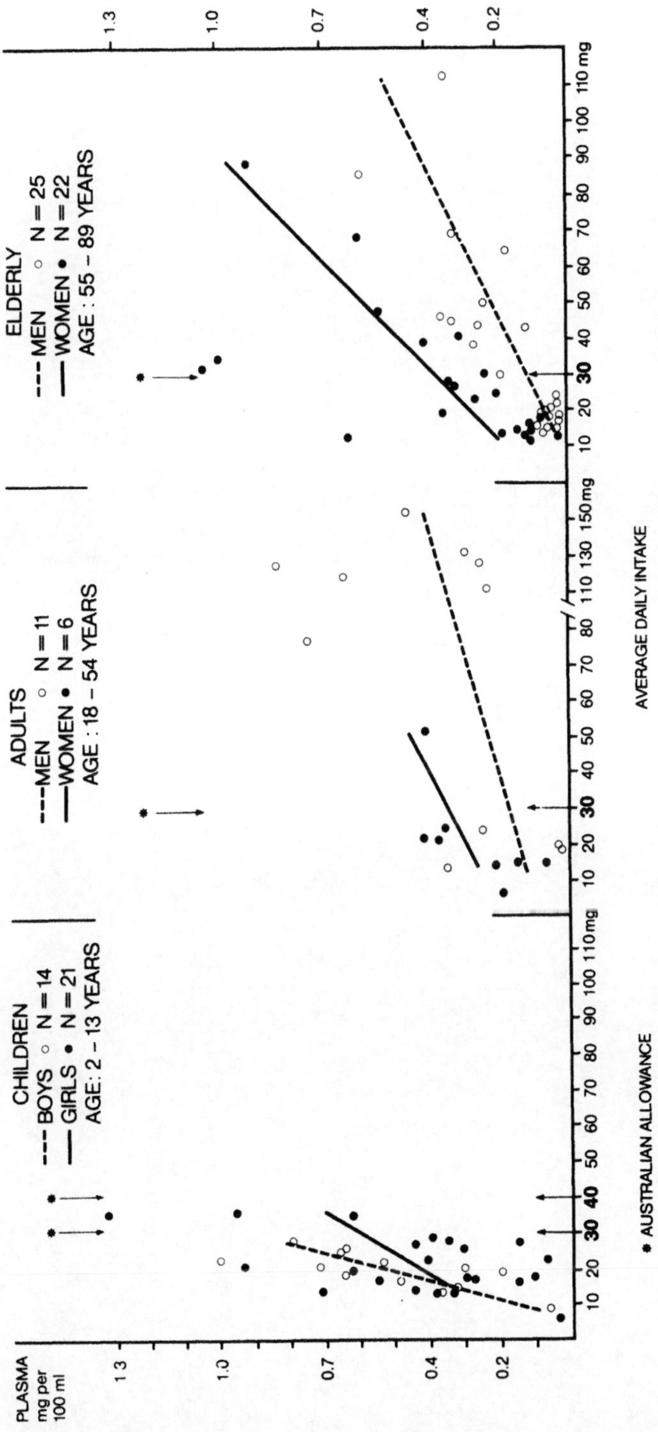

Figure 13 Vitamin C sex and age differences – intake versus plasma levels (from Woodhill (1979) with permission)

10
Vitamin C, modern lifestyle and hazards

Smoking and drinking, taking pills both prescribed or from self-medication, are all part of our modern lifestyle. Their effect on nutritional requirements in general and on vitamin C in particular is considerable. Not many studies have been undertaken to determine the mechanism by which these factors interfere with the metabolism of vitamin C.

10.1 VITAMIN C IN SMOKING AND HEAVY DRINKING

Smoking

Early and recent studies indicate that smokers have lower plasma and leukocyte levels of vitamin C than non-smokers (Irwin and Hutchins, 1976). Pelletier (1975) suggested that vitamin C absorption may be impaired in smokers and that smokers require more vitamin C than non-smokers to maintain similar blood levels of the vitamin. Ritzel (1974) reported a correlation between an increasing incidence of low plasma levels of vitamin C and an increasing number of cigarettes smoked daily; he compared non-smokers or limited smokers (0 to four cigarettes/day) with moderate smokers (five to 14 cigarettes/day) and heavy smokers (15 or more cigarettes/day). This trend was particularly marked in a group of 487 men aged 25 to over 65 years, whose diet did not include vitamin supplements, but was evident also in a group of 191 men who claimed to take vitamin preparations regularly. Ritzel (1974) suggested that acrolein, other unsaturated aldehydes or some oxidation product contained in tobacco could destroy ascorbic acid in the body. In their study with 178 healthy men aged 17–68 years McClean *et al.* (1976) reported that smokers in the youngest age group (17–29 years) had significantly lower plasma and leukocyte levels of vitamin C than non-smokers and that the younger smokers maintained the lower levels practically unaltered in later decades. These authors found no significant difference between the vitamin C levels of smokers and non-smokers in the age group 60–69 years, but noted that with increasing age plasma and leukocyte vitamin C appeared to decline in non-smokers. This study would support the view that young people should not take up smoking, and that old men require more vitamin C to withstand the ageing process.

Heavy drinking

Heavy drinkers are considered to be those people who consume regularly about 50 g alcohol per day. Anyone taking more than 80 g alcohol per day may easily become an alcoholic. All those who have measured vitamin C status in heavy drinkers seem to have found that vitamin C levels in the plasma or leukocytes are very low (see, for example, Baines, 1978). Whether this is due to poor dietary habits of alcoholics, liver involvement or direct effect of alcohol on vitamin C metabolism is not known (Bonjour, 1979). There are no studies on the effect of alcohol consumption below 50 g per day on vitamin C status. What happens to vitamin C in social drinking? The blood vitamin profile in scurvy from alcoholism was shown in Table 8. The subject (a 32-year-old man) had not only zero levels of vitamin C in the plasma but also deficient levels of vitamin A, the provitamin A (beta-carotene), vitamins B_1 and B_6. All levels appeared to have improved 16 days after daily administration of 300 mg ascorbic acid (Nobile, 1979).

10.2 VITAMIN C AND DRUGS

It is generally accepted that some drugs induce tissue desaturation of vitamin C. So far some investigations have been done on aspirin, oral contraceptives, iron, some anticonvulsants, antibiotics, antiobesity drugs and a few other drugs.

Aspirin

Aspirin and salicylates have been known for a long time to cause gastrointestinal haemorrhages. People can obtain aspirin easily without prescription and self-abuse is not uncommon. Loh and Wilson (1975) showed that intake of high doses of aspirin decreased plasma and leukocyte levels of vitamin C in normal healthy men. There seems to be a competition between the drug and ascorbic acid which causes a decreased uptake of ascorbic acid by the leukocytes. The drug is usually prescribed in the treatment of rheumatoid arthritis and other chronic inflammatory diseases. In these diseases body demands for vitamin C are increased and whenever aspirin is taken the therapy should include simultaneous administration of vitamin C (Loh and Wilson, 1975, Loh *et al.*, 1973).

Oral contraceptives

Briggs and Briggs (1974–75) reported that, amongst other vitamins, plasma vitamin C levels of 10 young healthy women on oral contraceptives were lower than in women who were not taking the drug. Treatment with high potency vitamin C and B-complex was reflected in higher plasma levels in the oral contraceptive group. Rivers (1975) found low plasma, leukocyte and platelet vitamin C levels in women on oral contraceptives but no decreased urinary excretion of the vitamin. He suggested that this effect may be due to the oestrogenic component of the pill and that there may be a change of ascorbic acid distribution in the tissues rather than a depletion of ascorbic acid reserves.

Other drugs

Several other drugs have been implicated in changes of vitamin C metabolism but much work must still be done to understand the interactions between vitamin C and drugs.

10.3 VITAMIN C AND CLIMATE

The effect of climate on the vitamin C requirements has been discussed by Irwin and Hutchins (1976). The issue appears to be controversial. The Russians (see Figure 9), for example, however recommend a double daily intake – in other words, 140 mg of vitamin C – for people living in the northern part of the country which is very cold.

11
Dietary recommendations for the healthy man and woman of the 1980s

It is known that animals perform better when they are well-nourished (Marks, 1975). Farmers and the owners of pet animals can purchase feeds containing specially prepared vitamin and mineral mixtures at concentrations suited to a particular animal species. The optimal vitamin requirements of cattle, sheep, horses, pigs, poultry, cats, dogs, etc. are well established . . . by man. Animals apparently thrive on them, and farm animals repay man by swelling his purse. Animals which can make vitamin C in their own bodies maintain its concentration in all tissues at so-called saturation levels. Why would they bother to do so if it were not necessary? Why should man not eat enough vitamin C to imitate the good example set by these animals? But what is enough for man?

The yo-yo of the dietary allowances of vitamin C recommended, for the healthy 'reference' individual of all ages, by various nutrition committees around the world is a result of work on the prevention and cure of overt scurvy in adults and not on optimal vitamin C requirements. What one needs to know is the vitamin C requirement of the infant, the growing child, the adult or elderly man and woman, not only to maintain their optimal health but also to aid in the restoration of their health when they are ill.

It is known that vitamin C functions in many metabolic pathways, that it is ubiquitous in active metabolic tissues and that it is a redox-system, giving up and receiving hydrogen ions. We recognize that vitamin C is a system comprising at least ascorbic acid, monodehydroascorbic acid and dehydroascorbic acid. It is not just one substance – ascorbic acid. It is accepted that vitamin C must be taken daily in the diet, that it is labile and can easily be destroyed by storage and cooking of food, or improper processing, or keeping meals hot after they are cooked. From our work with healthy adults it would seem that a daily intake of 67–130 mg vitamin C from food would ensure vitamin C levels in the plasma approaching tissue saturation, that is, ranging from 0.71 to 1.50 mg/100 ml. An intake of around 100 mg day vitamin C could be obtained easily by the inclusion in the daily diet of fruit and vegetables (see Appendix 2, page 139). We do not believe in the 10 mg minimal level of vitamin C intake, said to be sufficient to cure and prevent scurvy (Bartley, Krebs, and O'Brien, 1953, Baker *et al.*, 1969). We do not believe in the 30 mg dose, which is the allowance for vitamin C recommended in various countries, because this amount will maintain most individuals in a desaturation state (see Figures 7 and 12). The other extreme dose of 10 g advocated by Linus Pauling (1970) cannot be obtained from food only and will oversaturate the body with just one nutrient.

We believe that aiming at vitamin C intakes which would ensure levels in the plasma and body stores approaching tissue saturation is important for the maintenance of optimum state of health and better resistance to sudden physiopathological demands (Wilson, 1974). This advice was given in 1940 by Todhunter and Robbins (see page 89) and was confirmed in 1980 by the work of Kallner and his colleagues, who used labelled ascorbic acid to determine steady-state turnover and body pool of the vitamin in man.

We recommend, therefore, that helathy adult males and females eat a diet providing daily at least 70 mg of vitamin C if they do not drink or smoke regularly, and to double this intake if they are smokers, social or heavy drinkers and pill-takers (this includes women on oral contraceptives).

12
Ascorbic acid as a therapeutic agent – some controversial issues

In the preceding chapters we have discussed vitamin C as a nutrient, its chemistry, biochemical reactivity, its physiology or functions, and the vitamin C needs of the healthy person to ensure and maintain optimum wellbeing. Levels of vitamin C as high as 100 mg could easily be obtained daily from a balanced diet made up of foods commonly used; to attain this goal there is no need to resort to pills and potions.

In the treatment of scurvy, which is a vitamin C-specific disease, doses of the vitamin varying between 200 and 2000 mg are needed daily, depending on the speed at which tissue resaturation is required (Marks, 1975). Doses of vitamin C, in grams, which exceed the amounts present in the usual diet, have to be taken in the form of ascorbic acid or its salts, sodium ascorbate and calcium ascorbate. Ascorbic acid is the reducing moiety of the redox-system of vitamin C which is available commercially in tablets or other pharmaceutical preparations or as the crystalline material. Used in this way ascorbic acid is considered a therapeutic agent and prescribed medically for the treatment of the specific disease, scurvy.

In recent years the use of ascorbic acid as a therapeutic agent has been proposed and investigated for the treatment of other diseases such as the common cold, viral infections, atherosclerosis, cancer, and psychiatric disorders. The efficacy of high doses of ascorbic acid in the prevention and cure of these diseases has been neither proved nor disproved. The issue is controversial and some of the aspects of the controversy will be discussed in the following sections.

It must be emphasized that, in contrast to other drugs, ascorbic acid is part of the vitamin C system. It is a nutrient, a physiologically consonous substance, which is stored and circulates in the human body and is essential for metabolic functions of the tissues and which, by its physicochemical nature, is a very labile and very reactive compound.

12.1 ASCORBIC ACID AND THE COMMON COLD

What is the common cold?

The common cold, or acute rhinitis, is an inflammation of the upper respiratory tract caused by a viral infection. It is an acute and highly contagious, infectious disease. Miller and Keane (1972) stated that at least 20 identifiable viruses had been found to cause colds and in 1974 Merigan reported that the number of viruses known to be responsible for the common cold is about 100. The incidence of the common cold has been estimated at about three colds per person per year (Pauling, 1970). According to Canadian statistics, 'the disability from acute (mainly respiratory) illness amounts to approximately 1.5 days per person per year. In terms of total personal income (approximately 66 billion dollars in 1970) this is equivalent to a loss of approximately 270 million dollars annually' (Anderson, Reid, and Beaton, 1972).

The common cold may develop if a person is exposed to low temperature conditions and/or to an infected atmosphere that may be produced by a person with a cold, who sneezes bacteria and viruses into the air (Lewin, 1976). The development of the symptoms of a cold is dependent upon the state of health and environmental factors (Pauling, 1970). Tyrrell (1965) reported that the symptoms develop when a particular virus–host relationship occurs, and Wilson (1971) claimed that the host tissue must be in a susceptible state for the attack by the virus. It is agreed that the period of incubation, that is, the time between exposure and occurrence of the symptoms, is usually 2–3 days and that the first symptom is often a scratchy and sore throat.

Miller and Keane (1972) state that

> all colds are not identical, because of different causative agents and individual reactions. Usually the common cold starts with a runny nose, sneezing, a stuffy feeling in the head, slight headache, watering of the eyes, general aching and listlessness, inability to concentrate and perhaps a slight fever. The affected membranes swell until the nasal passages are blocked. Often the inflammation spreads to the throat, causing sore throat and cough. The senses of smell and taste are blunted so that the patient hardly knows or cares what he is eating. He has no energy or ambition and just wants to lie down, as in fact he should.

Anderson, Reid, and Beaton (1972) classified the symptoms of a cold as respiratory, those affecting either the nose, throat or chest, and non-respiratory such as malaise, chills and attacks of gastroenteritis. Wilson and Loh (1973) proposed a distinction between toxic symptoms (headache, fever, malaise, sore throat) and catarrhal symptoms (headcold, cough, nasal obstruction, nasal discharge). A cold may last from 7 to 14 days, and may be followed by serious complications such as laryngitis, bronchitis, pneumonia, sinus infection, infection of the middle-ear, and exacerbation of other diseases (Miller and Keane, 1972). The traditional treatment is: resting in bed at the first sign of a cold, and keeping warm; avoiding exposure to temperature changes and to irritants such as smoking; drinking fruit juices, hot lemon drinks and water; eating a simple but nutritious diet; and alleviating the symptoms by taking drugs such as aspirin. No specific drugs had been suggested for the *prevention* of the common cold until ascorbic acid was used as both a prophylactic and therapeutic agent.

Ascorbic acid and the common cold

We have reviewed 92 references, covering the period from 1942 to 79 on the use of ascorbic acid for the prevention and treatment of the common cold (see Section 15.1). Among these references there are six monographs, 34 descriptions of trials on the effect of ascorbic acid on the common cold, and three on its effect on viral infection, 22 reports on vitamin C metabolism in the common cold, four editorials, seven letters to the editor, four review articles; the remaining 12 are comments on various aspects of the problem. Dated between 1942 and 1969 are 14 trials on the common cold, one study on viral infection, one editorial and one monograph; all remaining 75 articles appeared in the literature after the publication of Linus Pauling's book *Vitamin C and the Common Cold* in 1970.

The 37 trials on ascorbic acid and its effect on the common cold and viral infection were conducted in several countries: the United States, Canada, England and Scotland, Eire, Australia, Scandinavia, Belgium and Switzerland. The subjects studied were drawn from the general population or from selected groups such as schoolchildren, adolescents, postgraduate and university students, marine recruits, personnel of companies, prisoners, skiers, medical personnel, and medical practitioners and their families. The type of control was either single-blind or double-blind. The duration of the experiments varied between 2½ days and 5 years. The daily dose of ascorbic acid used as a supplement during the trials ranged from 195 mg to 10 g. The vitamin was administered in the form of either syrup, powder, tablets, effervescent preparations or sustained-release capsules containing either ascorbic acid and/or its sodium or calcium salts. In some trials ascorbic acid was either added to orange juice or administered in conjunction with multivitamin tablets. The control group usually received a placebo preparation. Few investigators commented on the vitamin C content and the type of the diet which the subjects consumed either before or during the experiment; few investigators measured vitamin C levels in the blood plasma, white blood cells or urine to determine vitamin C status (see Chapter 9) of the subjects before, during and after the trial. The majority of the investigators assumed that the subjects selected were in good health, and did not differentiate between the subjects' age and sex. In most of the trials, the method of assessment of the incidence, type, duration and severity of the colds was based on the subjects' self-records. Statistical evaluation of the results was measured by relating appearance, duration and severity of the symptoms of the colds to the dose of ascorbic acid. The results of these trials are conflicting. Lewin (1976) has summarized 19 trials, as illustrated in Table 12, and we have adopted his classification to evaluate the results of the 37 trials which we have reviewed:

(1) no benefit – nine trials
(2) some benefits but mainly no benefit – five trials
(3) some benefits – five trials
(4) beneficial effects – 18 trials.

(1) Ascorbic acid had *no beneficial effects* on the prevention of colds when viruses were inoculated directly into the nose and the throat (Walker, Bynoe, and Tyrrell, 1967), in the prophylaxis of induced rhinovirus 44 infection (Schwartz *et al.*, 1973), and in acute illness of the upper respiratory tract (Coulehan *et al.*, 1975; 1976). The effects of ascorbic acid on the common cold were considered of no benefit by six groups of investigators (Dahlberg, Engel, and Rydin, 1944; General Practitioner Trials, 1968; Glazebrook and Thomson, 1942; Pitt and Costrini, 1979; Tebrock, Arminio, and Johnston, 1956; Tyrrell *et al.*, 1977).

(2) *Some benefits but mainly no benefit* were reported in five studies (Cowan, Diehl, and Baker, 1942; Elwood *et al.*, 1976; Elwood, Hughes, and St. Leger, 1977; Lewis *et al.*, 1975; Ludvigsson, Hansson, and Tibbling, 1977).

(3) *Some beneficial effects* of ascorbic acid on the reduction of the number of colds and of the number of days off work were obtained in five trials (Anderson *et al.*, 1975; Anderson, Reid, and Beaton, 1972; Caels, 1953; Karlowski *et al.*, 1975; and Miller *et al.*, 1977).

(4) *Beneficial effects* on the incidence, type, duration and severity of the symptoms of colds from different doses of ascorbic acid were reported in 18 trials (Anderson, Suranyi, and Beaton, 1974; Baird *et al.*, 1979; Banks, 1968; Barnes, 1961; Broadhurst and Crafter, 1975; Charleston and Clegg, 1972; Cheraskin *et al.*, 1973; Clegg and MacDonald, 1975a,b; Colby *et al.*, 1974; Coulehan *et al.*, 1974; Dietz, 1957; Franz, Sands, and Heyl, 1956; Markwell, 1947; Regnier, 1968; Ritzel, 1961; Wilson and Loh, 1969b, 1973).

Biochemical and molecular biological aspects of vitamin C and the common cold

Wilson and his colleagues in Eire, and Lewin in England, are the first and appear to be the only workers who investigated, biochemically and at the molecular level, the fate of vitamin C in the human body affected by the common cold. Wilson's group and Lewin recognized that there are wide variations between indi-

Table 12 Effect of vitamin C on the common cold and allied respiratory malaises (Lewin, 1976)

Investigators and year	*Type of participants*	*Daily dose (g)*	*Type of control (blind)*	*Ascorbate or ascorbic acid*	*Tablets or powder*	*Ascorbate content of blood*	*Attackers determination bacteria viruses*	*Interpretation*
Cowan, Diehl, and Baker (1942)	students	0.2–0.5	single-blind	acid	tablets	—	c.c	slight benefits, mainly no benefit
Glazebrook and Thomson (1942)	adolescents	up to 0.2	—	acid	powder or tablets	—	c.c.	practically no benefit
Markwell (1947)	general population	0.75	—	acid	n.s.	—	c.c.	beneficial
Caels (1953)	general population	10	—	acid	syrupy solution	—	c.c.	some benefit (general wellbeing)
Franz, Sands, and Heyl (1956)	medical students and nurses	3×0.065	single-blind	acid	capsules	determined	c.c.	beneficial
Ritzel (1961)	adults (skiers)	1:0	single-blind	acid	tablets	—	c.c.	beneficial
Barnes (1961)	high school pupils	0.2	—	n.s.	multivitamin tablets	—	c.c.	multivitamin tablets with vitamin C: beneficial
Banks (1965)	personnel of firms	n.s.	double-blind	n.s.	capsules	—	c.c.	beneficial
Walker, Bynoe, and Tyrrell (1967)	adults	3.0	single-blind	effervescent	tablets	—	several viruses inoculated	
Regnier (1968)	general population	0.6. every 3 hr	double/single-blind	ascorbic acid	powder	—	c.c.	beneficial
General practitioner trials (1968)	medical practitioners and families	3×1	double-blind	effervescent	tablets	—	c.c.	no benefit
Anderson, Reid, and Beaton (1972)	general population	1.0	double-blind	ascorbate	tablets	—	c.c.	some benefit
Charleston and Clegg (1972)	students and lecturers	1.0	single-blind	—	tablets	—	—	beneficial
Cheraskin *et al.* (1973)	medical practitioners and wives	0.2–0.4		n.s.	n.s.	—	c.c.	beneficial
Schwartz *et al.* (1973)	adult male prisoners	3×1	double-blind	acid	tablets	determined	rhinovirus 44	no benefit
Wilson and Loh (1973)	boys and girls schools and students	0.2–0.5	single-blind	acid	tablets	determined	c.c.	beneficial
Coulehan *et al.* (1974)	school children	1 and 2	double-blind	acid	tablets	determined	c.c.	beneficial
Anderson, Suranyi, and Beaton (1974)	general population	0.25–8	double-blind	ascorbate	tablets	—	c.c.	beneficial at highest doses
Karlowski *et al.* (1975)	adults	3–6	mainly double-blind	ascorbate	capsules	—	c.c.	some benefit

n.s. = not stated
c.c. = common cold

viduals in their physiological requirements for vitamin C and that pathological conditions such as the common cold greatly affect vitamin C requirements. They further recognized that age, sex and the degree of vitamin C saturation have significant effects on vitamin C metabolism in the tissues.

Biochemical aspects – studies in Eire

Wilson and his colleagues (Greene and Wilson, 1975; Loh and Wilson, 1970, 1971a,b,c,d; Wilson, 1971; 1973c; 1974; 1975a, b,c,d,e; 1976a,b; Wilson and Greene, 1978; Wilson and Loh, 1969b; 1973; Wilson, Loh, and Foster 1973a,b; Wilson, Greene, and Loh, 1976) conducted trials on vitamin C and the common cold with schoolchildren and university students of both sexes, with the following results:

(1) They observed that cold symptoms may be of a toxic or a catarrhal nature or a combination of both, and that there is a sex difference in the complexity and frequency of these symptoms. Boys tended to have more complex symptoms than girls, and girls tended to have colds that are more intense and of longer duration than boys.
(2) They studied vitamin C metabolism and storage by measuring plasma, white blood cell levels, and urinary excretion of vitamin C before, during and after a cold.
(3) They showed that there is an association between susceptibility to colds and abnormalities of vitamin C metabolism. They demonstrated that supplementary ascorbic acid during the winter months raised significantly tissue levels of vitamin C in subjects susceptible to cold viruses, and significantly reduced duration, severity and incidence of cold symptoms in adolescents.
(4) They established a way by which cold symptoms can be related to vitamin C storage and metabolism by evaluating the changes in plasma and white blood cell levels before, during and after a cold. They reported a significant positive correlation between metabolic utilization of vitamin C during colds and the severity of cold symptoms.
(5) They observed that during the first 3 days of the common cold, white blood cell stores of vitamin C were significantly

reduced in both sexes (an observation confirmed by Hume and Weyers, 1973); plasma levels of vitamin C tended to be lower and urinary excretion of the vitamin was diminished. With the development of the viral infection, the vitamin C stores in the white blood cells decreased further as the vitamin leached out into the plasma. Plasma levels were thus increased, ready for transport to the tissues infected and particularly to the respiratory tissues when catarrhal symptoms occurred. The passage of vitamin C from white blood cells into the plasma, and hence to the tissues in need, was more pronounced in males than in females during a cold.

(6) They administered a single dose of 500 mg of ascorbic acid during the first 3 days of a cold and observed that 6 hours after the administration plasma levels of vitamin C were increased, but little vitamin C was excreted in the urine, and white blood cell levels were still low both in males and females. However, 3 weeks after disappearance of all symptoms, plasma and white blood cell levels were increased but more significantly in females than in males. When, at this stage (3 weeks after recovery from a cold), a 500 mg dose of ascorbic acid was administered, repletion of vitamin C stores as indicated by vitamin C moving from the plasma into the white blood cells, was significantly greater in females than in males. This indicated that the 500 mg dose of ascorbic acid was sufficient, for the females, to resaturate the tissues which were depleted during the common cold, while in the males tissue desaturation was still present. The authors reported that a prophylactic dose of 500 mg of ascorbic acid daily could significantly reduce the intensity of upper respiratory infections in females but was not effective in males.

(7) They increased the load dose up to 2000 mg ascorbic acid and observed that, 4 hours after the administration, white blood cell levels were significantly increased in the women but only slightly in the men.

(8) They reported that maintenance of tissue saturation by a *therapeutic dose* of 2000 mg ascorbic acid at the onset of a cold and every 6 hours was associated with reduction in severity of cold symptoms in the acute stage of a cold.

In reviewing the work of his unit, Wilson (1974) reported that alterations of vitamin C metabolism occur in other respiratory diseases and in antigen–antibody reactions. Vitamin C is needed in the white blood cells to ensure phagocytosis and to aid in reformation of mucous membranes which are destroyed during the common cold. It may also act in preventing replication of RN (ribonucleic acid) and DNA (deoxyribonucleic acid) in bacteriophage viruses. He pointed out that bleeding of the nose, pains in the joints and muscles, and mental depression, which often occur during the acute stages of a cold, are typical symptoms of scurvy – that is, of vitamin C deficiency.

Wilson and his colleagues do not recommend lifelong intakes of megadoses of ascorbic acid. They emphasize the need to ensure that intakes of vitamin C in the diet are sufficient to maintain tissue saturation and stores at all times in the healthy person so that sudden physiopathological demands may be met. The common cold is an example of a sudden physiopathological demand which may deplete vitamin C stores; if this happens, to prevent the development of cold symptoms appropriate doses of supplementary vitamin C should be taken to restore and maintain the leukocyte levels at saturation.

More supplementary ascorbic acid may be needed by men than by women and a prophylactic daily dose of 2000 mg of vitamin C can be expected to prevent the onset of a cold in 80 to 90% of the population, irrespective of sex. The continuation of such treatment, once the stores of vitamin C in the white blood cell levels are repleted and health is restored, is unjustified and may, in the long run, have adverse effects (Wilson, 1974, see Section 12.6).

Vitamin C and the common cold: its molecular biology – studies in England

Molecular biology is 'the study of the biochemical and biophysical aspects of structure and function of genes and other subcellular entities, and of such specific proteins as haemoglobins, enzymes and hormones; it provides knowledge of cellular differentiation and metabolism and of comparative evolution' (Miller and Keane, 1972). Lewin (1976) published a book which includes an extensive bibliography on various aspects and problems of vitamin C. In this book Lewin reported that with the development of a cold there is a *progressive malfunctioning of physiological activities*. He stated that the common cold may develop if a person is exposed (a) to low temperatures, and (b) to an infected atmosphere.

Exposure to low temperature conditions

The respiratory system is chilled and the results are a 'disordered hormone balance followed in a vicious circle by decreased levels of the cyclic nucleotide adenosine 3′,5′-monophosphate (cAMP) [see Sections 3.2 and 6.2], decreased antibody and interferon production'. Under such conditions the bacteria and viruses, originally quiescent in the respiratory tract, can attack freely and a cold would develop. The attack is likely to be overcome, however, if high levels of vitamin C are present in the blood and in the respiratory tract *in time* to prevent a decrease of cAMP (Lewin, 1974b,c; 1976; Tisdale, 1975) and thus to ensure increased resistance to the bacteria and viruses.

Exposure to an infected atmosphere (as produced, for example, by sneeze droplets)

In such a case the activity of the respiratory membranes and of other membranes, as well as enzyme formation, become disorganized, hormone balance is disturbed and the vicious circle, mentioned in the preceding paragraph, follows. Here again, if vitamin C is present in high doses in the *early stages* of the viral attack, it could contain it and inhibit depression of cAMP levels. Vitamin C acts in these cases through the formation of the monodehydroascorbic acid free radical (MDHAA) which, however, requires the presence of oxygen; if catarrhal symptoms develop, aeration is limited and the formation of the free radical MDHAA is inhibited.

Lewin stressed the importance of the *time* factor in initiating the intake of ascorbic acid. He recommends 1 g doses as soon as a cold threatens to develop and stresses the need to continue such an intake at intervals of approximately 1½ hours. This treatment would ensure attainment and maintenance of maximum concentration of the vitamin in the respiratory system, in the white blood cell and other defence mechanisms and tissues, *in time* to withstand the viral attack. Most human tissues, including the lungs and the mucous membranes, normally store vitamin C in levels higher than those of blood plasma where the vitamin is present only for active transport (see Table 4, page 62). High vitamin C levels in the blood and in the respiratory system are needed to inhibit hydrolytic destruction of cAMP by phosphodiesterase, and thus to maintain the cAMP levels required for adequate physiological activity (see Sections 3.2 and 6.2). Lewin (1976) reports that, *in vitro*, ascorbic acid has been shown to be a more efficient inhibitor of cAMP phosphodiesterase than other drugs such as aspirin and codeine (Moffat *et al.*, 1972).

It is of interest to note that there seems to be consensus of opinion that vitamin C also acts as an antihistamine.

Comments on trials

All reviewers review trials in the light of their own expertise. We are very aware of the problem of dietary assessment and interrelationship of nutrients and particularly vitamins. If vitamin C is to be considered as a therapeutic agent, all the factors affecting vitamin C status of the subjects must be quantitated before statistical correlations can be attempted. Some of the measurements, such as dietary intakes, will be crude but vitamin C intake must be related to calories, fibre, alcohol and to all nutrients. Measurement of vitamin C in blood plasma (transport), white blood cells (stores) and urine (excretion) can and must be done in any trial or study designed to demonstrate the therapeutic effect of ascorbic acid. The interactions and interrelationships of vitamin C with other nutrients (protein, carbohydrates, fat, vitamins and minerals), with drugs, smoking and alcohol can be studied by laboratory measurements. Several disease conditions are known to affect vitamin C status; thus screening for disease should be included in the description of subjects admitted into a clinical trial.

We have documented the attempts of research workers to test whether or not ascorbic acid is effective in preventing the common cold, and whether or not it has an influence on the duration and severity of the symptoms. Of 37 trials quoted 18 have reported benefits; some of the investigators were able to establish a statistical significance for these benefits. Other investigators (for example, Coulehan, 1979) imply that 'the benefits shown are probably due to statistical artifacts, minor vitamin C-induced physiological changes, the placebo effect or a combination of these'. Anderson (1977) advocates the need for further large-scale, and strictly double-blind, trials. To us it seems unlikely that large-scale trials on vitamin C and the common cold will provide a satisfactory answer to its beneficial or non-beneficial effects on the single or complex symptoms of the common cold, because it is almost impossible to plan clinical trials which will take into account all the variables related to this problem, such as:

(1) individual variation in the susceptibility to viral infections which may have a genetic basis and may be sex-dependent;
(2) variation in the symptoms of the common cold and problems associated with the measurement of these symptoms;
(3) variation in the type of viruses;
(4) variation of the vitamin C content of tissues and blood levels depending upon age and sex;
(5) individual variation in vitamin C metabolism, which may have a genetic basis or may be due to dietary habits, smoking or pill-taking, past or present disease conditions, not only those involving the respiratory system.

Other variables are:

(1) As vitamin C is interrelated with many nutrients, it is important to ascertain whether or not the diet is adequate in calories, fibre, all nutrients, not only in vitamin C; and whether or not the dietary pattern is distorted by high intakes of sugar, fat and alcohol.
(2) Smoking, oral contraceptives and aspirin are known to affect vitamin C metabolism, but the effect of other drugs is not known and all pill-takers should be excluded from a trial.
(3) Vitamin C is interrelated with many nutrients and metabolites but the precise role and relationship is not known. Measurement of all possible biochemical and haematological parameters should be made before the trial, daily during the attacks of the common cold and after all symptoms have disappeared. The tests should include measurement of minerals such as iron, copper and magnesium, functional tests for the vitamins B_1, B_2 and B_6 and plasma levels of all other vitamins, not only vitamin C.
(4) Vitamin C levels of the selected subjects in the test group and the control group should be measured in blood plasma,

white blood cells and urine. The urine tests should include measurement of the intact ascorbic acid and of its metabolites.

(5) Attempts should be made to relate the results to cAMP (cyclic adenosine 3′,5′-monophosphate) levels and/or to the inhibition of phosphodiesterase during the experimental period (Lewin, 1976).

(6) The effect of substances which may be contained in the placebo preparation should be eliminated and account should be taken of the time/diet factors which can have a controlling role in the protection or destruction of ascorbic acid in the gastrointestinal tract.

(7) Precautions should be taken to ensure that any factor affecting ascorbic acid stability in the supplement is eliminated.

(8) It should be ensured that the ascorbic acid is taken *in time* at the sign of the very first symptoms or whenever the subject came in contact with a person affected by a cold.

Summary

Vitamin C is a very labile compound and a very reactive and important redox-system; this means that it is constantly active in either giving up or receiving hydrogen. It must be ubiquitous as it is found in every tissue which has high metabolic activity including the lungs and the respiratory system. One of the main functions of vitamin C is to maintain the integrity of the membranes.

It is documented that in certain stress conditions tissue levels of vitamin C are decreased. As long as the conditions are reasonably homeostatic the redox-system is in equilibrium but when stress, trauma, pathological conditions, or attack by viruses occur, the system is disturbed. The reaction pushes further towards excess utilization of vitamin C through oxidation, hydrolysis and other unknown processes. The vitamin is no longer active and is destroyed; its fine physicochemical reversible reactivity is out of kelter.

We accept that these conditions justify the use of high doses of ascorbic acid for a short time as a therapeutic agent to prevent the development of the common cold and to shorten its duration.

Questions

(1) *Does ascorbic acid prevent the onset of a cold?*
We consider it may, if *taken in time* at the first scratchiness of the throat or other early symptoms and after contact with persons with a cold.

(2) *Does ascorbic acid reduce duration and severity of the symptoms?*
Evidence from several trials points in this direction.

(3) *How much ascorbic acid is needed for prevention of a cold and reduction of its duration and severity?*
It depends on the state of tissue saturation. Research workers in this field have suggested that a therapeutic dose of 1–2 g, if taken at the very first symptoms and at 6 hour intervals for 1–2 days may suffice for most people to prevent the onset of a cold. They suggest further that the dose should be repeated until the symptoms disappear. Then it is recommended to reduce the dose gradually to avoid a sudden drop of vitamin C blood levels.

(4) *Is ascorbic acid in high dosages harmful?*
There is no evidence to show that it is harmful if taken for the prevention of colds or for the duration of a cold which may last 7–14 days.

(5) *What harm could come from the habitual intake of ascorbic acid in 1 g or higher doses?*
There is no evidence to suggest that the healthy person needs to continue to take megadoses of ascorbic acid (that is, more than ten times the amount needed to maintain tissue saturation). If for any reason high doses of ascorbic acid are prescribed, it would be advisable to take it in the form of multivitamin–multimineral preparations to avoid nutrient and metabolic imbalance. Side-effects have to be considered and a high level of intake of one nutrient may throw out of gear many of the finely adjusted physiological mechanisms of body metabolism.

12.2 ASCORBIC ACID AND CANCER

Vitamin C status as measured by plasma and leukocyte levels is impaired in patients with malignant disease (Kakar, Wilson, and Bell, 1975; Kakar, Wilson and Moriarty, 1977), so the requirement is high. As ascorbic acid is a strong reducing agent, and is involved in many metabolic reactions, it may interfere with the metabolism of neoplastic cells. The studies carried out in recent years indicate that ascorbic acid may be effective in controlling and preventing cancer. This may be attributed to its ability to potentiate the protective mechanism in the body rather than to a specific anticancer effect (Pauling, 1979).

12.3 ASCORBIC ACID AND ATHEROSCLEROSIS

The lesion in coronary heart disease has been studied in relation to vitamin C nutrition by Ginter *et al.* (1979). In subjects with mild or moderate hypercholesterolaemia and low vitamin C status, administration of ascorbic acid considerably affected cholesterol levels. If hypercholesterolaemia is the result of chronic imbalance between exogenous and endogenous cholesterol, therapy with ascorbic acid has hopes of succeeding. Willis, Light, and Gow (1954) and Spittle (1973) described therapeutic effects of ascorbic acid in atherosclerosis and vascular thrombosis, but the hypothesis that cholesterol from atheromas is mobilized by vitamin C requires experimental verification (Ginter *et al.*, 1979).

12.4 ASCORBIC ACID AND OTHER DISEASES

As our literature survey indicates ascorbic acid has been used in the therapy of various diseases, sometimes successfully, sometimes not. This is not surprising, firstly, because one should determine vitamin C status of the patients, and secondly, because the function of vitamin C is not yet clarified.

12.5 ASCORBIC ACID IN SURGICAL TRAUMA

It is common practice today to prepare a patient for operation by prescribing adequate vitamin C and other vitamins. A recent report by Irvin, Chattopadhyay, and Smythe (1978) suggests that surgical intervention resulted in an increased ascorbic acid requirement.

12.6 MEGADOSES OF ASCORBIC ACID

Megadose is a term which has become fashionable in the context of vitamin supplementation. The prefix 'mega' used in this sense means 'large', and not one million as when it refers to a specific unit of measurement (such as megavolt). The term megadose seems to have jelled solely to vitamins as we do not hear it applied to mineral or protein supplementation.

Any substance may have side-effects if taken in excess of certain limits, which may vary from individual to individual. In the case of ascorbic acid, megadoses are regarded as gram-doses which are not attainable from food. The side-effects of any therapeutic agent have to be balanced against its usefulness and the urgency of treating a disease. To our knowledge there were no known drugs which could prevent the onset of the common cold until ascorbic acid was tried and found useful, at least by some people and some investigators. The common cold is a disease which fortunately does not last long but which may have some nasty consequences. If large doses of ascorbic acid can prevent the onset of the common cold, it is better to take it, and to take it *in time*, and *as much as is needed*, rather than to have to resort when the cold has developed to all sort of drugs, pills and potions, which are not physiologically consonous and may themselves have harmful effects. But once the cold has subsided, there is *no valid reason* to continue the ascorbic acid treatment. Our advice is: do not drop the high dosage of ascorbic acid suddenly, but drop it gradually and then return to a vitamin C-rich diet, balanced with all the other nutrients.

Megadoses of ascorbic acid for the treatment of diseases such as atherosclerosis and cancer is another aspect of therapy which medical practitioners may prescribe; they have to balance the pros and cons of megadoses of ascorbic acid against the pros and cons of other drugs.

Many studies have been conducted to test whether or not megadoses of ascorbic acid have harmful effects on the human organism. So far the results are conflicting and the issue is still controversial. Side-effects from megadoses of ascorbic acid which have been reported in the literature are as follows:

Gastrointestinal disturbances

Some individuals may have diarrhoea and excessive gas formation after large intakes of ascorbic acid (Anderson, Reid, and Beaton, 1972). This can be prevented by taking the vitamin with meals or with methylcellulose (Lewin, 1976).

Acidosis

Acidosis means the accumulation of acid or depletion of alkaline reserves in blood or body tissues. Ascorbic acid has been prescribed for many years as an agent to acidify the urine in doses as high as 3–6 g per day. It has been shown that although ascorbic acid can lower the pH of urine, the effect on the pH of blood was negligible (Barness, 1975; Lewin, 1976).

Interaction with other nutrients

The following points should be noted:

(1) High doses of ascorbic acid should not be taken in a low-protein, high-carbohydrate diet as the protein is essential in preventing undesirable high levels of dehydroascorbic acid and glucose in the blood. This was reported by Chatterjee's group in 1975.

(2) Vitamin C and vitamin B_{12} work together in the treatment of megaloblastic anaemia (Terroine, 1966). Herbert and Jacob (1974) and Herbert *et al.* (1978) claimed, from an *in vitro* experiment, that the vitamin B_{12} content of blood is destroyed if doses of ascorbic acid higher than 0.5 g are taken with meals. Other workers (such as Afroz *et al.*, 1975; Marcus *et al.*, 1980) could not reproduce this finding and demonstrated that the claim was due to inadequacy of the extraction method used.

(3) If the diet is low in copper and zinc, high doses of ascorbic acid may increase the mineral deficiency (Barness, 1975).

(4) High levels of sugar in blood and urine (hyperglycaemia and hyperglycosuria) have been attributed to megadoses of ascorbic acid until it was discovered that the claim was due to analytical ignorance. Ascorbic acid, like sugar, is a reducing agent and enhances the reaction of sugars by reducing the reagents normally used for testing urine and blood sugar. When this fact was realized and appropriate modifications of the test were introduced, the claim was demonstrated to be untenable (Barness, 1975; Lewin, 1976).

Oxaluria (increased oxalate in urine)

It is known that about 50% of the daily excretion of oxalic acid in the urine comes from the catabolism of vitamin C. Oxalic acid is formed when metabolic oxidation of ascorbic acid proceeds beyond the dehydroascorbic acid stage. It is known that ingestion of ascorbic acid in daily doses up to 4 g produces only a slight increase in urinary oxalate but in doses of 4 g and above the increase becomes more marked (Barness, 1975; Lewin, 1976).

Renal calculi (kidney stones)

It is known that there are individuals who are prone to stone formation such as oxalate stones, uric acid stones and cystine stones. It has been inferred that high doses of ascorbic acid would accelerate the formation of such stones. So far only one case of a healthy individual developing a urinary *oxalate* stone after ingestion of ascorbic acid for a short time has been reported (Briggs, Garcia-Webb, and Davies, 1973). Barness (1975) stated that he could find no report of oxalate stone formation in normal individuals who had no enzymatic defects and we could find no references to such a claim in the literature up to the end of 1979. It has been shown that urinary excretion of uric acid increases when high doses of ascorbic acid are taken, but the increase in *uric acid* levels in the blood is minimal (Lewin, 1976) or nil (Stein, Hasan, and Fox, 1976). Stein and his colleagues in 1976 found that high doses of ascorbic acid had no effect on protein-bound uric acid. These authors stated that ascorbic acid could invalidate studies involving measurement of uric acid and obscure the diagnosis of gout, and that, *theoretically*, it could precipitate gouty arthritis or renal calculi in predisposed persons. So far no reports have been found in the literature to relate *cystine* stones to ascorbic acid.

Ascorbic acid is known to act as a diuretic (Lewin, 1976), which means that it would facilitate urinary flow and decrease the probability of stone formation. Could this not be the reason why more oxalic acid and uric acid are found in the urine after ingestion of large doses of ascorbic acid? Could it be that ascorbic acid does facilitate their excretion rather than promote the formation of oxalate and uric acid stones? Moreover, ascorbic acid is an acid, and the excess of requirement by the tissues is excreted in the urine as ascorbic acid intact, so the urine becomes more acid and calcium oxalate would dissolve in this medium as it is more soluble in acid than in alkaline solutions (Lewin, 1976). Ascorbic acid is used in large doses in the treatment of spinally injured patients to acidify their urine because it can form salts with sodium (Na), calcium (Ca), ammonium (NH_4) etc. Has anybody investigated whether these patients have ever developed kidney stones?

Interference with drugs

Patients who are being treated with anticoagulants (warfarin, dicoumarol) should not be taking megadoses of ascorbic acid because it could shorten the prothrombin time. This has been rarely observed (Barness, 1975; Lewin, 1976).

Infertility and infant scurvy

Some investigators have claimed that megadoses of ascorbic acid favour infertility or abortion, but others who have prescribed up to 10 g/day of ascorbic acid to several patients failed to observe such an effect (Lewin, 1976). Cochrane (1965) attributed scurvy which developed in two young infants to the high doses of ascorbic acid that the mothers took during their pregnancies. No other report on this was found in the literature.

Withdrawal syndrome

When a person has been taking megadoses of ascorbic acid for a long period, the body may have become conditioned to the 'de-luxe' treatment, in other words, to using the vitamin at a high level. Sudden withdrawal of the treatment does not allow the physiology of the individual to accommodate immediately to a lower intake. He is still, in effect, working in high gear and quickly uses up all available reserves of the vitamin. As a result the body pools of vitamin C are rapidly depleted and scurvy may be precipitated. Although only some investigators (Schrauzer and Rhead, 1973, for example) have reported this finding, the physiological rationale may be explained because ascorbic acid is a very reactive and very mobile substance. Other investigators have failed to observe such a result so that here again individual variability may play a role. It is advisable, therefore, to reduce the doses gradually in order to allow the body to readapt to the lower intake of the vitamin and to avoid complications.

Interference of ascorbic acid in the assay of glucose, uric acid and other biochemical parameters

An analyst must be aware that any method he uses for testing a particular substance is bound to have some limitations. There are many substances which interfere in the assay of vitamin C in foods and in human and animal tissues (sugar is one of them); it is not surprising that the interference is reciprocal. Interference of ascorbic acid with autoanalyser assays of serum transaminase, lactic dehydrogenase and bilirubin has been reported (Barness, 1975). The first report of the Expert Group on 'drug interference in clinical chemistry' of the Bureau of Reference, Directorate General for Research, Science and Education of the Commission of the European Communities (Siest *et al.*, 1978) stated that ascorbic acid, in therapeutic concentrations, had no influence on the analytical values of urea, cholesterol, calcium, protein, bilirubin (see above), aspartate, aminotransferase and alkaline phosphatase, but it did interfere with the assay of glucose, uric acid, creatinine and inorganic phosphate. The interference was found to vary depending on the type of reaction and the apparatus used. In some case the interference of ascorbic acid was such that the values of other parameters were useless. An experienced analyst, *au fait* with modern techniques, can modify methods to eliminate interferences.

Summary

Common sense indicates that the healthy person should avoid the habitual excessive intake of just one nutrient, as this will cause nutrient imbalance which sooner or later may result in some serious metabolic disturbances. Even if the results of the various studies are conflicting and even if one authority states that the side-effects of megadoses of ascorbic acid are 'insignificant, rare or troublesome but of little consequence' (Barness, 1975), it is advisable that megadoses of ascorbic acid are not taken by individuals who are prone to stone formation, by patients on anticoagulant therapy and by pregnant women. But neither should they take too little vitamin C.

13
Vitamin C and future research

As we have indicated in this book, there are many gaps in the knowledge of vitamin C. We have attempted to summarize in a schematic form what is known and what is still unknown about nutritional interrelationships (Figure 14), metabolic interactions of vitamin C (Figure 15), the effects of modern lifestyle and everyday hazards on vitamin C requirements (Figure 16), and vitamin C in various diseases of mankind (Figure 17).

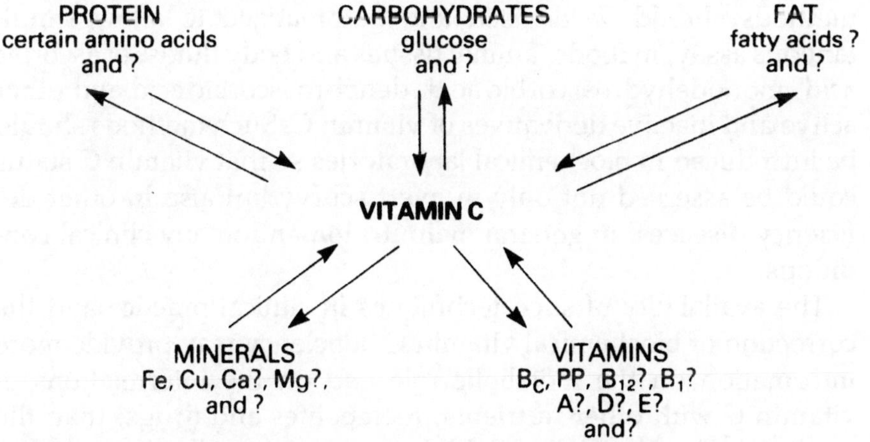

Figure 14 Nutritional interrelationships of vitamin C

We have stressed that vitamin C is a redox-system comprising at

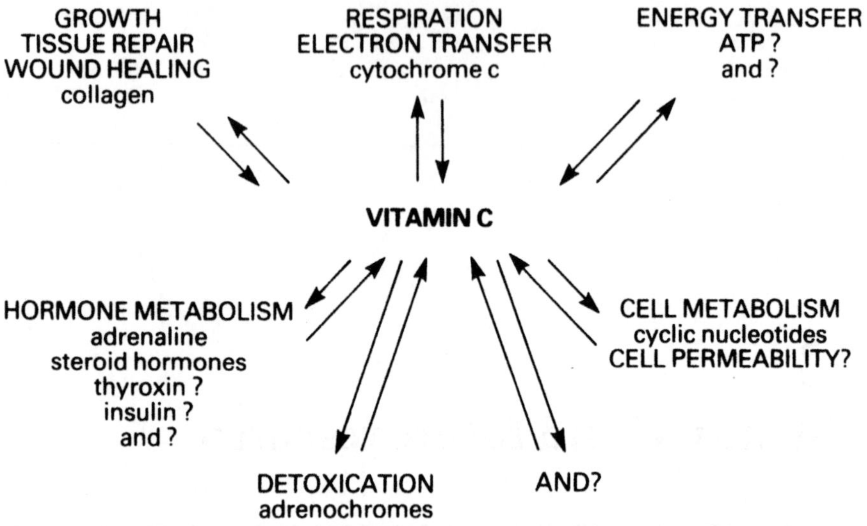

Figure 15 Metabolic interaction of vitamin C

least three substances: L-ascorbic acid, monodehydro-L-ascorbic acid and dehydro-L-ascorbic acid. We believe that research into the role of the redox-system in itself and its components, not just of ascorbic acid alone, will be more helpful in discovering the exact function of vitamin C in human metabolism. As long as the precise function of vitamin C remains a mystery, no functional test can be developed to determine vitamin C status. Meanwhile analytical methods should be devised and automatized to allow simultaneous assay, in foods, animal tissues and body fluids, of ascorbic acid, monodehydroascorbic acid, dehydroascorbic acid and other active and inactive derivatives of vitamin C. Such methods should be introduced in biochemical laboratories so that vitamin C status could be assessed not only in overt scurvy but also in other deficiency diseases, in general malnutrition and in any clinical conditions.

The availability of such techniques in clinical practice and the correction of biochemical vitamin C deficiency may provide more information on the metabolic role and on the interrelations of vitamin C with other nutrients, metabolites and drugs, than the study of vitamin C in healthy persons. Longitudinal studies should be undertaken to determine the importance of keeping vitamin C at approaching tissue saturation levels to maintain

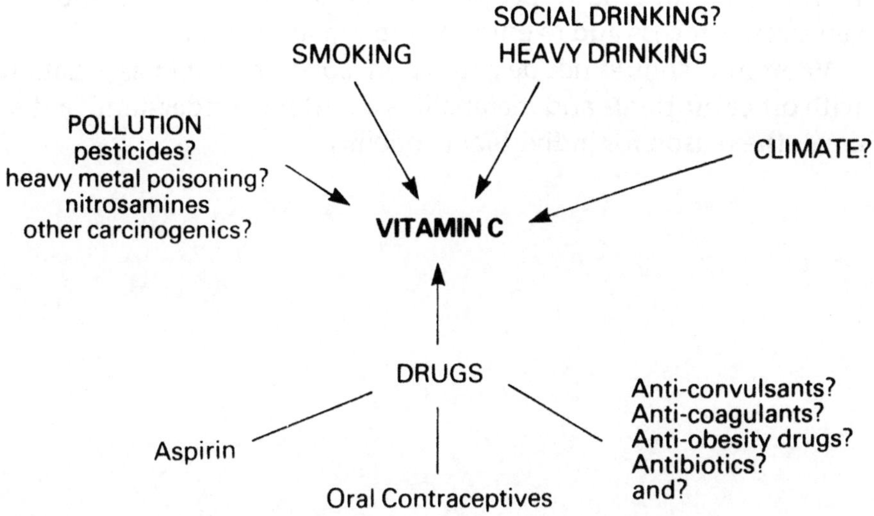

Figure 16 Vitamin C and modern lifestyle and hazards

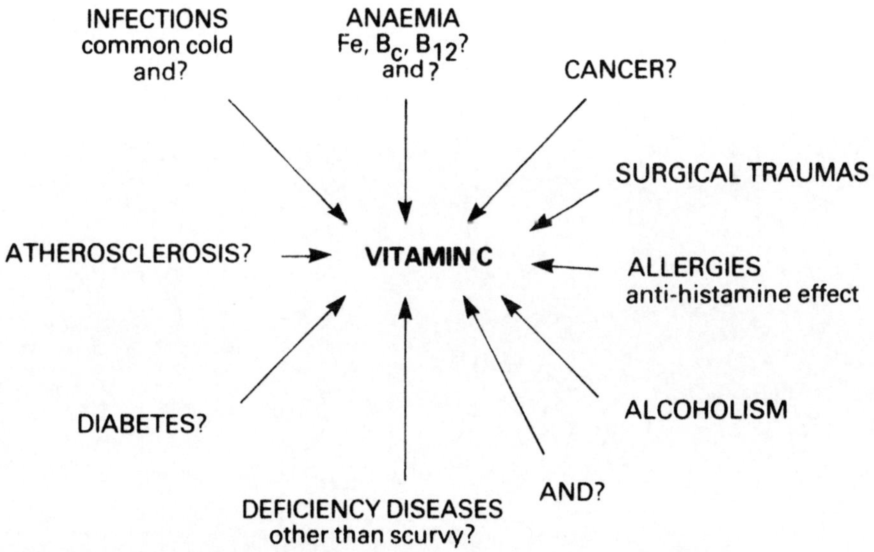

Figure 17 Vitamin C and diseases

optimum health and improve resistance to disease. These studies will provide a basis for assessing vitamin C requirements in children, adolescents, pregnant and lactating women, and adult and elderly males and females. Maintenance of tissue saturation levels of vitamin C in elderly people may help them to withstand the senescent process and to enjoy a better quality of life.

Vitamin C should not be studied in isolation, but in association with other nutrients and metabolites in order to understand or discover the reason for individual variability.

14
Appendix 1
Summary of the fluorimetric determination of vitamin C in blood plasma

Heparinized blood

▼

Centrifuge
5 minutes at 2500 rpm

▼

Plasma
(0.5–2 ml)

▼

Stabilization and deproteinization
1 ml plasma and 9 ml 5% HPO_3. Shake 1 minute and store at −20°C

▼

Thaw at RT, **Centrifuge**
5 minutes at 2500 rpm

▼

Oxidation
2 ml clear extract + 10 μl0.1 N Iodine. Mix, after 10 seconds add 5 μl 0.5 N $Na_2S_2O_3$. Mix again. Divide the oxidized extract into 3 test tubes (a, b, c).

▼

Buffering

	Test (l)		*Blank* (ml)
	a	*b*	*c*
Oxidized extract	0.5	0.5	0.5
Sodium acetate 25% aq.	0.5	0.5	—
Sodium acetate 25% aq. +10% boric acid	—	—	0.5

Mix, let stand 15 min at RT in the dark

▼

Condensation to fluorescent quinoxaline

Add 0.2 ml *o*-Phenylene diamine dihydrochloride 0.1% aq. to each of the 3 test tubes (a), (b) and (c)

Mix, let stand 15 min at RT in the dark

▼

Fluorimetric measurement

(interference filters excitation 366 nm, emission 423 nm). Set instrument with quinine sulphate 0.1 μg/ml in 0.1 N H_2SO_4 and read samples immediately

▼

Calculation

from calibration curve of L-ascorbic acid after correction of fluorescence reading for blank.

Vitamin C (mg/100 ml plasma)

Clinical deficiency	0–0.20
Biochemical deficiency	0.21–0.40
Marginal status	0.41–0.70
Acceptable levels (tissue saturation levels)	0.71–1.50

Appendix 2
Examples of daily menus providing adequate vitamin C

To evaluate your daily menus for vitamin C:

(1) write down everything you eat and drink for one day,

(2) underline all the foods you expect to contain vitamin C,

(3) look up Table 3, and sum up the total vitamin C content: you should have at least 70 mg of vitamin C per day, that is, at least 4.5 vitamin C points per day.

TYPICAL BRITISH MENU (ABOUT 2000 CALORIES/DAY)

	Quantity of food*	*Calories*	*Vitamin C mg*	*Vitamin C points*
Breakfast				
Orange juice, fresh	100 ml	38	50	3.5
Porridge, oatmeal	60 g	26	0	0
Milk	150 ml	see below		
Sugar	20 g	see below		
Toast, 1 slice	30 g	see below		
Butter	10 g	see below		
Marmalade	25 g	65	2.5	
Tea, 2 cups				
Milk	60 ml	see below		

* For the purpose of this calculation it is sufficiently accurate to consider that 1 g ≃ 1 ml

	Quantity of food*	*Calories*	*Vitamin C mg*	*points*
Midmorning coffee				
Coffee, 2 cups				
Milk	60 ml	see below		
Biscuits	10 g	46	0	0
Lunch				
Sandwiches				
Bread, 2 slices	60 g	see below		
Corned beef	25 g	60	0	0
Pickles, sweet	25 g	34	0	0
Butter	15 g	see below		
Cake, madeira	50 g	196	0	0
Apple, 1 with peel	100 g	46	5	0.5
Tea				
Milk	60 ml	see below		
Midafternoon coffee				
Coffee, 2 cups				
Milk	60 ml	see below		
Whisky and soda				
Whisky, 2 nips	50 g	111	0	0
Soda				
Dinner				
Clear tomato soup	200 g	10	10	0.5
Roast, sirloin	100 g	284	0	0
Horseradish sauce	5 g	3	6	0.5
Gravy	10 g	10	0	0
Yorkshire pudding	50 g	108	0	0
Roast potatoes	50 g	78	2.5	
Peas, boiled, fresh	50 g	26	7.5	0.5
Carrots, boiled	50 g	10	2	
Stewed prunes, with sugar	50 g	52	0	0
Milk pudding rice	100 g	131	0	0
Cream, whipped	30 g	100	0.3	
Milk	30 ml	see below		
Coffee				
Total				
Milk	420 ml	273	2.1	
Sugar	20 g	79	0	0
Bread, wholemeal	90 g	194	0	0
Butter	25 g	185	0	0
	Total	2165	87.9	5.5

VEGETARIAN MENU (ABOUT 2000 CALORIES/DAY)

	Quantity of food*	*Calories*	*Vitamin C mg*	*Vitamin C points*
Breakfast				
Orange juice, fresh	100 ml	38	50	3.5
Muesli	25 g	92	0	0
Milk	150 ml	see below		
Sugar	20 g	see below		
Toast, 1 slice	30 g	see below		
Butter	10 g	see below		
Marmalade	25 g	65	2.5	
Lunch				
Lentils, boiled	100 g	99	0	0
Tomato, raw, sliced	100 g	14	20	1.5
Spring greens, boiled	100 g	10	30	2
Apple, 1 with peel	100 g	46	5	0.5
Dried apricots	50 g	91	0	0
Bread, 2 slices	60 g	see below		
Butter	20 g	see below		
Milk	100 ml	see below		
Dinner				
Cheese	50 g	155	0	0
Eggs, 2	100 g	147	0	0
Potatoes, new, boiled	100 g	76	18	1
Peas, boiled, fresh	100 g	52	15	1
Prunes, stewed with sugar	50 g	52	0	0
Milk pudding rice	100 g	131	0	
Bread, 1 slice	30 g	see below		
Butter	10 g	see below		
Milk	100 ml	see below		
Total				
Milk	350 ml	228	1.75	
Sugar	20 g	79	0	0
Bread, wholemeal, 4 slices	120 g	259	0	0
Butter	40 g	296	0	0
	Total	1930	142.25	9.5

* For the purpose of this calculation it is sufficiently accurate to consider that 1 g $\simeq$ 1 ml

ITALIAN MENU (ABOUT 2000 CALORIES/DAY)

	Quantity of food*	*Calories*	*Vitamin C mg*	*Vitamin C points*
Breakfast (prima colazione)				
Bread roll, 1, crusty white	50 g	see below		
Butter	10 g	see below		
Jam or orange marmalade	15 g	39	1.5	
Coffee, 2 large cups				
Milk	200 ml	see below		
Sugar	30 g	see below		
Morning coffee				
Coffee, 1 small cup				
Sugar	10 g	see below		
Midday dinner (*colazione o pranzo*)				
Risotto (boiled rice)	100 g	123	0	0
with fish, cooked	50 g	48	0	0
oil	5 g	see below		
Chicken, roast	50 g	108	0	0
Peas, fresh, boiled	50 g	26	7.5	0.5
Salad, mixed, green	100 g	12	15	1
Oil	5 g	see below		
Apple, 1 with peel	100 g	46	5	0.5
Bread roll, 1 crusty white	50 g	see below		
Wine (*vino*)	200 ml	see below		
Afternoon coffee				
Coffee, 1 small cup				
Sugar	10 g	see below		
Evening meal (*cena*)				
Spaghetti, boiled	150 g	175	0	0
Meat, mince	50 g	114	0	0
Tomato paste	10 g	7	10	0.5
Oil	5 g	see below		
Salad, mixed, green	100 g	12	15	1
Oil	5 g	see below		
Spinach, boiled	100 g	30	25	1.5
Fruit, 1 orange	100 g	35	50	3.5
Bread roll, 1, crusty white	50 g	see below		
Wine (*vino*)	200 ml	see below		

* For the purpose of this calculation it is sufficiently accurate to consider that 1 g $\simeq$ 1 ml

	Quantity* of food	Calories	Vitamin C mg	points
Total				
Milk	200 g	130	1	
Sugar	50 g	197	0	0
Bread rolls, 3, crusty white	150 g	435	0	0
Butter	10 g	74	0	0
Oil	20 g	180	0	0
Wine (*vino*)	400 ml	300	0	0
	Total	2091	130	8.5

15
References

Afroz, M., Bhothinard, B., Etzkorn, J.R., Horenstein S. and McGarry, J.D. (1975). Letter: Vitamins C and B_{12}. *J. Am. Med. Assoc.*, **232(3)**, 246

Anderson, T.W. (1975). Large scale trials of vitamin C. *Ann. NY Acad. Sci.*, **258**, 498

Anderson, T.W. (1977). Large scale studies with vitamin C. *Acta Vitaminol. Enzymol. (Milano)*, **31(1–5)**, 43

Anderson, T.W., Reid, D.B.W. and Beaton, G.H. (1972). Vitamin C and the common cold. A double-blind trial. *Can. Med. Assoc. J.*, **107**, 503

Anderson, T.W., Suranyi, G. and Beaton, G.H. (1974). The effect on winter illness of large doses of vitamin C. *Can. Med. Assoc. J.*, **111**, 31

Attwood, E.C., Robey, E.D., Ross, J., Bradley, F. and Kramer, J.J. (1974). Determination of platelet and leucocyte vitamin C and the levels found in normal subjects. *Clin. Chim. Acta*, **54**, 95

Baines, M. (1978). Detection and incidence of B and C vitamin deficiency in alcohol-related illness. *Ann. Clin. Biochem.*, **15(6)**, 307

Baird, I.M., Hughes, R.E., Wilson, H.K., Davies, J.E.W. and Howard, A.N. (1979). The effects of ascorbic acid and flavonoids on the occurrence of symptoms normally associated with the common cold. *Am. J. Clin. Nutr.*, **32(8)**, 1686

Baker, E.M. (1967). Vitamin C requirements in stress. *Am. J. Clin. Nutr.*, **20**, 583

Baker, E.M., Hodges, R.E., Hood, J., Sauberlich, H.E. and March, S.C. (1969). Metabolism of ascorbic-1-^{14}C acid in experimental human scurvy. *Am. J. Clin. Nutr.*, **22(5)**, 549

Baker, E.M., Hodges, R.E., Hood, J., Sauberlich, H.E., March, S.C. and Canham, J.E. (1971). Metabolism of ^{14}C and ^{3}H-labelled L-ascorbic acid in human scurvy. *Am. J. Clin. Nutr.*, **24**, 444

Ball, E.G. (1937). Studies on oxidation-reduction. XXIII. Ascorbic acid. *J. Biol. Chem.*, **118**, 219

Banerjee, S. (1977). Physiological role of dehydroascorbic acid. *Indian J. Physiol. Pharmacol.*, **21(2)**, 85

Banks, H.S. (1968). Controlled trials in the early antibiotic treatment of colds. *Med. Officer*, **119**, 7

Barkhan, P. and Howard, A.N. (1958). Distribution of ascorbic acid in normal and leukaemic human blood. *Biochem. J.*, **70**, 163

Barnes, F.E. (1961). Vitamin C supplements and the incidence of colds in High School basketball players. *N.Carolina Med. J.*, **22,** 22
Barness, L.A. (1975). Safety considerations with high ascorbic acid dosage. *Ann. NY Acad. Sci.*, **258,** 523
Bartley, W., Krebs, H.A. and O'Brien, J.R.P. (1953). Vitamin C requirements of human adults. Special Report Series Medical Research Council, London. No. **280,** 1–179
Bermond, P. and Rilliet B. (1975). Statut vitaminique d'un groupe de sujets hospitalisés ou fréquentant une policlinique. In G. Brubacher and G. Ritzel (eds.), *Zur Ernährungssituation der schweizerischen Bevölkerung*, pp.178–200
Bezssonoff, M.N. and Woloszyn, M. (1938). Sur l'existence d'une forme oxydée intermediaire entre la vitamine C et l'acide dehydroascorbique. *Bull. Soc. Chim. Biol.*, **20,** 93
Bielski, B.H.J., Richter, H.W. and Chan, P.C. (1975). Some properties of the ascorbate free radical. *Ann. NY Acad. Sci.*, **258,** 231
Bogdanov, N.G. and Zviagina, O.P. (1975). Bound forms of ascorbic acid combined with the blood serum proteins. *Vopr. Pitan*, **(6),** 24 (Russian). English Abstract.
Bonjour, J.P. (1979). Vitamins and alcoholism. I. Ascorbic acid. *Int. J. Vit. Nutr. Res.*, **49(4),** 434
Booth, J.B and Todd, G.B. (1970). Subclinical scurvy–hypovitaminosis C. *Br. J. Hosp. Med.*, **4,** 513
Bourges, H., Chavez, A. and Arroyo, P. (1970). *Recomendaciones de Nutrimentos para la Poblacion Mexicana.* Publicacion L-17 de la Division de Nutricion. Instituto Nacional de Nutricion, Mexico.
Briggs, M.H., Garcia-Webb, P. and Davies, P. (1973). Urinary oxalate and vitamin C supplements. *Lancet*, **2,** 201
Briggs, M. and Briggs, M.H. (1974–75). Changes in biochemical indices of vitamin nutrition in women using oral contraceptives during treatment with Surbex 500. *Curr. Med. Res. Opin.*, **2(10),** 626
British Medical Association (1950). *Report of the Committee on Nutrition.* (London: British Medical Association)
Broadhurst, N.A. and Crafter, K.C. (1975). Vitamin C and the common cold. *Austr. Family Physician*, **4 (April),** 271, 275, 277
Burns, J.J. (1961). Vitamin C. *Ann. NY Acad. Sci.*, **92,** 1
Caels, F. (1953). Contribution a l'étude de l'effet de hautes doses de vitamine C dans les infections oto-rhino-laryngologiques. *Acta Oto-Rhino-Laryngol. Belg.*, **7,** 395
Charleston, S.S. and Clegg, K.M. (1972). Ascorbic acid and the common cold. *Lancet*, **1,** 1401
Chatterjee, G.C. (1967). Biochemical detection of deficiency. In W.H. Sebrell, Jr. and R.S. Harris, *The Vitamins, 2nd. Edition, Vol. 1*, pp. 399–407. (New York: Academic Press Inc.)
Chatterjee, I.B., Kar, N.C., Ghosh, N.C. and Guha, B.C. (1961). Aspects of ascorbic acid biosynthesis in animals. *Ann. NY Acad. Sci.*, **92,** 36
Chatterjee, I.B., Majumder, A.K., Nandi, B.K. and Subramanian, N. (1975). Synthesis and some major functions of vitamin C in animals. *Ann. NY Acad. Sci.*, **258,** 24
Cheraskin, E., Ringsdorf, W.M., Michael, D.W. and Hicks, B.S. (1973). Daily vitamin C consumption and reported respiratory findings. *Int. J. Vit. Nutr. Res*, **43,** 42
Clegg, K.M. and MacDonald, J.M. (1975a). L-ascorbic acid and D-isoascorbic acid

in a common cold survey. *Am. J. Clin. Nutr.*, **28(9)**, 973

Clegg, K.M. and MacDonald, J.M. (1975b). D-isoascorbic acid investigated in a common cold survey. *Proc. Nutr. Soc.*, **34(1)**, 7A

Cochrane, W.A. (1965). Overnutrition in prenatal and neonatal life: A problem? *Can. Med. Assoc. J.*, **93**, 893

Colby R.H., Brown, J., Fine, R. and Karlson, R. (1974). Quoted by S. Lewin (1974a)

Coulehan, J.L. (1979). Ascorbic acid and the common cold: reviewing the evidence. *Postgrad. Med.*, **66(3)**, 153, 157, 160.

Coulehan, J.L., Resinger, K.S., Rogers, K.D. and Bradley, D.W. (1974). Vitamin C prophylaxis in a boarding school. *N. Engl. J. Med.*, **290**, 6

Coulehan, J.L., Kapner, L., Eberhard, S., Taylor, F.H. and Rogers, K.D. (1975). Vitamin C and upper respiratory illness in Navaho children: preliminary observations (1974) *Ann. NY Acad. Sci.*, **258**, 513

Coulehan, J.L., Eberhard, S., Kapner, L., Taylor, F., Rogers, K. and Garry, P. (1976). Vitamin C and acute illness in Navajo school children. *N. Engl. J. Med.*, **295(18)**, 973

Cowan, D.W., Diehl, H.S. and Baker, A.B. (1942). Vitamins for the prevention of colds. Maximum dose of 500 mg vitamin C. *J. Am. Med. Assoc.*, **120**, 1267

Crandon, J.H., Lund, C.C. and Dill, D.B. (1940). Experimental human scurvy *N. Engl. J. Med.*, **223**, 353. In Sebrell, W.H. Jr. and Harris, R.S. (1967). *The Vitamins, 2nd. Edition, Vol.1.* (New York: Academic Press Inc.)

Dahlberg, G., Engel, A. and Rydin, H. (1944). The value of ascorbic acid as a prophylactic against 'common colds'. *Acta Med. Scand.*, **119**, 540.

Dawson, C.R., Strothkamp, K.G. and Krul, K.G. (1975). Ascorbate oxidase and related copper proteins. *Ann. NY Acad. Sci.*, **258**, 209

Department of Health and Social Security (1969). *Recommended Intakes of Nutrients for the United Kingdom. Report on Public Health and Medical Subjects 120.* (London: HMSO)

Department of Health and Social Security (1979). *Recommended Daily Amounts of Food Energy and Nutrients for Groups of People in the United Kingdom. Report on Health and Social Subjects 15.* (London: HMSO)

Derman, D.P., Bothwell, T.H., MacPhail, A.P., Torrance, J.D., Bezwoda, W.R., Charlton, R.W. and Mayet, F.G.H. (1980). Importance of ascorbic acid in the absorption of iron from infant foods. *Scand. J. Haematol.*, **25**, 193

Deutsch, M.J. and Weeks, C.E. (1965). Microfluorometric assay for vitamin C. *J. Assoc. Off. Agr. Chem.*, **48**, 1248

Dietz, N. Jr. (1957). The common cold and stress conditions. *Indust. Med. Surg.*, **26(5)**, 229

Dodds, M.L. (1969). Sex as a factor in blood level of ascorbic acid. *J. Am. Diet. Assoc.*, **54**, 32

Drummond, J.C. (1920). In H.R. Rosenberg (1945). *Chemistry and Physiology of the Vitamins.* (New York: Interscience Publishers, Inc.)

Elger, K. (1980). Trustee *Commonsense Cookery Book.* Cookery Teachers Association of New South Wales. Early editions 1906, 1912. Personal communication.

Elwood, P.C., Lee, H.P., St.Leger, A.S., Baird, M. and Howard, A.N. (1976). A randomized controlled trial of vitamin C in the prevention and amelioration of the common cold. *Br. J. Prev. Soc. Med.*, **30(3)**, 193

Elwood, P.C., Hughes, S.J. and Leger, A.S. (1977). A randomized controlled trial of the therapeutic effect of vitamin C in the common cold. *Practitioner*, **218(1303)**, 133

Fazio, V.A., Wahlqvist, M.L. and Flint, D. (1979). Ascorbic acid status in nu-

tritionally vulnerable groups. MSc thesis submitted at Deakin University, Geelong
Floridi, A., Coli, R., Fidanza, F., Bourjois, C.F. and Wiggins, R.A. (1981). High pressure liquid chromatographic determination of ascorbic acid in food: comparison with other methods. *Int. J. Vit. Nutr. Res.*, **51**, (in preparation)
Food and Agriculture Organisation of the United Nations (FAC/WHO) (1970). *Requirements of Ascorbic Acid, Vitamin D, Vitamin B_{12}, Folate, and Iron.* Report of a Joint FAO/WHO Expert Group. FAO No. 47 and WHO No. 452. Rome
Franz, W.L., Sands, G.W. and Heyl, H.L. (1956). Blood ascorbic acid level in bioflavonoid and ascorbic acid therapy of common cold. *J. Am. Med. Assoc.*, **162,** 1224
Funk, K. (1912). In H.R. Rosenberg (1945). *Chemistry and Physiology of the Vitamins.* (New York: Interscience Publishers, Inc.)
Gehler, J. and Kubler, W. (1970). Verteilungsstudien mit intravenös infundierter Ascorbinsäure. *Int. Z. Vitaminforsch.*, **40,** 454
General Practitioner Trials (1968). Ineffectiveness of vitamin C in treating coryza. *Practitioner*, **200,** 442
Ginter, E., Bobek, P., Babala, J., Jakubovský, J., Zaviačič, M. and Lojda, Z. (1979). Vitamin C in atherosclerosis. In A. Hanck and G. Ritzel (eds.) *Vitamin C.* Suppl.19 to *Int. J. Vit. Nutr. Res.*, pp. 55–70. (Bern: Hans Huber Verlag)
Glazebrook, A.J. and Thomson, S. (1942). The administration of vitamin C in a large institution and its effect on general health and resistance to infection. *J. Hyg.*, **42(1),** 1
Greene, M. and Wilson, C.W. (1975). Effect of aspirin on ascorbic acid metabolism during colds (proceedings). *Br. J. Clin. Pharmacol.*, **2(4),** 369P
Gyorgy, P. (ed.) (1950). *Vitamin Methods, Vol. 1*, p. 287. (New York: Academic Press Inc.)
Heath, H. (1962). The distribution and possible functions of ascorbic acid in the eye. *Exp. Eye Res.*, **1,** 362
Herbert, V. and Jacob, E. (1974). Destruction of vitamin B_{12} by ascorbic acid. *J. Am. Med. Assoc.*, **230(2),** 241
Herbert, V., Jacob, E., Wong, K.T., Scott, J. and Pfeffer, R.D. (1978). Low serum vitamin B_{12} levels in patients receiving ascorbic acid in megadoses: studies concerning the effect of ascorbate on radioisotope vitamin B_{12} assay. *Am. J. Clin. Nutr.*, **31(2),** 253
Hodges, R.E., Baker, E.M., Hood, J., Sauberlich, H.E. and March, S.C. (1969). Experimental scurvy in man. *Am. J. Clin. Nutr.*, **22(5),** 535
Howells, G., Palmer, P.E.S. and St. John-Brooks, W.H. (1954). Six cases of infantile scurvy. *Br. Med. J.*, **Nov. 13,** 1143
Hume, R. and Weyers, E. (1973). Changes in leucocyte ascorbic acid during the common cold. *Scot. Med. J.*, **18,** 3
Interdepartmental Committee on Nutrition for National Defense (1963). *Manual for Nutrition Surveys. 2nd. edition* (Bethesda, Md: National Institutes of Health)
Interdepartmental Committee on Nutrition for National Defense. Nutrition survey reports (1957–1971). Washington, DC
Irvin, T.T., Chattopadhyay, D.K. and Smythe, A. (1978). Ascorbic acid requirements in postoperative patients. *Surg. Gynecol. Obstet.*, **147,** 49
Irwin, M.I. and Hutchins, B.K. (1976). A conspectus of research on vitamin C requirements of man. *J. Nutr.*, **106(6),** 823
Jolliffe, N. (1959). *Current Concepts of Nutrition. I. Nutritional Deficiency Disease – Pathogenesis and Diagnosis.* Medical Research, Lederle, American Cyanamid Company, USA, p. 6

Jolly, M. and Nobile, S. (1977). Vitamin status of patients with oral lichen planus. *Aust. Dent. J.*, **22(6)**, 446

Kakar, S.C., Wilson, C.W.M. and Bell, J.N. (1975). Plasma and leucocyte ascorbic acid concentrations in acute lymphoblastic leukaemia. *Irish J. Med., Sci.*, **144(6)**, 227

Kakar, S.C., Wilson, C.W.M. and Moriarty, M.J. (1977). The relationship between cancer, radiotherapy and vitamin C. *Irish J. Med. Sci.*, **146(9)**, 289

Kallner, A., Hartmann, D. and Hornig, D. (1977a). Determination of bodypool size and turnover rate of ascorbic acid in man. *Nutr. Metab.*, **21 (Suppl. 1)**, 31

Kallner, A., Hartmann, D. and Hornig, D. (1977b). On the absorption of ascorbic acid in man. *Int. J. Vit. Nutr. Res.*, **47(4)**, 383

Kallner, A., Hartmann, D. and Hornig, D. (1979). Steady-state turnover and bodypool of ascorbic acid in man. *Am. J. Clin. Nutr.*, **32**, 530

Kamien, M., Nobile, S., Cameron, P. and Rosevear, P. (1974). Vitamin and nutritional status of a part Aboriginal community. *Aust. NZ J. Med.*, **4**, 126

Kamien, M., Woodhill, J.M., Nobile, S., Cameron, P. and Rosevear, P. (1975a). Nutrition in the Australian Aborigines – effects of the fortification of white flour. *Aust. NZ J. Med.*, **5**, 123

Kamien, M., Woodhill, J.M., Nobile, S., Rosevear, P., Cameron, P. and Winston, J.M. (1975b). Nutrition in the Australian Aborigine. *Food Technol. Aust.*, **27(3)**, 93

Karlowski, T.R., Chalmers, T.C., Frenkel, L.D., Kapikian, A.Z., Lewis, T.L. and Lynch, J.M. (1975). Ascorbic acid for the common cold. A prophylactic and therapeutic trial. *J. Am. Med. Assoc.*, **231(10)**, 1038

Kern, M.I. and Racker, E. (1954). Activation of DPNH oxidase by an oxidation product of ascorbic acid. *Arch. Biochem. Biophys.*, **48**, 235

King, C.G. (1975). Current status of vitamin C and future horizons. *Ann. NY Acad. Sci.*, **258**, 540

Kinsman, R.A. and Hood, J. (1971). Some behavioral effects of ascorbic acid deficiency. *Am. J. Clin. Nutr.*, **24**, 455

Levin, E.Y., Levenberg, B. and Kaufman, S. (1960). The enzymatic conversion of 3,4-dihydroxyphenylethlyamine to norepinephrine. *J. Biol. Chem.*, **235**, 2080

Lewin, S. (1974a). Vitamin C and the common cold. Abbreviated report of the 1973 international conference held in Stanford. *Chem. Br.*, **10(1)**, 25

Lewin, S. (1974b). The use of megaquantities of ascorbic acid or ascorbate for therapeutic and prophylactic purposes in relation to biochemical individuality. *Biochem. Soc. Trans.*, **2**, 154

Lewin, S. (1974c). The ascorbate system and the formation of adenosine 3′:5′-cyclic monophosphate. *Biochem. Soc. Trans.*, **2**, 400

Lewin, S. (1976). *Vitamin C: Its Molecular Biology and Medical Potential.* (London, New York, San Francisco: Academic Press)

Lewis, T.L., Karlowski, T.R., Kapikian, A.Z., Lynch, J.M., Shaffer, G.W., George, D.A. and Chalmers, T.G. (1975). A controlled clinical trial of ascorbic acid for the common cold. *Ann. NY Acad. Sci.*, **258**, 505

Loh, H.S. and Wilson, C.W.M. (1970). The origin of ascorbic acid stored in the leucocytes. *Br. J. Pharmacol.*, **40**, 169P

Loh, H.S. and Wilson, C.W.M. (1971a). An improved method for the measurement of leucocyte ascorbic acid concentrations. *Int. J. Vit. Nutr. Res.*, **41**, 90

Loh, H.S. and Wilson, C.W.M. (1971b). Relationship between leucocyte and plasma ascorbic acid concentrations. *Br. Med. J.*, **3**, 733

Loh, H.S. and Wilson, C.W.M. (1971c). The relationship between leucocyte ascorbic acid and haemoglobin levels at different ages. *Int. J. Vit. Nutr. Res.*, **41**, 259

Loh, H.S. and Wilson, C.W.M. (1971d). The relationship between leucocyte ascorbic acid concentrations and total white cell blood count. *Int. J. Vit. Nutr. Res.*, **41,** 253

Loh, H.S. and Wilson, C.W.M. (1975). The interactions of aspirin and ascorbic acid in normal men. *J. Clin. Pharmacol,* **15(1),** 36

Loh, H.S., Watters, K. and Wilson, C.W.M. (1973). The effects of aspirin on the metabolic availability of ascorbic acid in human beings. *J. Clin. Pharmacol.*, **13 (11 and 12),** 480

Lowry, O.H. (1952). Biochemical evidence of nutritional status. *Physiol. Rev.*, **32,** 431. In W.H. Sebrell, Jr. and R.S. Harris, (1967). *The Vitamins 2nd. Edition, Vol.1.* (New York: Academic Press Inc.)

Lowry, O.H., Bessey, O.A. and Burch, H.B. (1952). Effects of prolonged high dosage with ascorbic acid. *Proc. Soc. Exp. Biol. Med.*, **80,** 361. In Sebrell, W.H. Jr. and Harris, R.S. (1967). *The Vitamins, 2nd Edition, Vol. 1,* p. 404. (New York: Academic Press Inc.)

Ludvigsson, J., Hansson, L.O. and Tibbling, G. (1977). Vitamin C as a preventive medicine against common colds in children. *Scand. J. Infect. Dis.*, **9(2),** 91

Mapson, L.W. (1956). Losses of vitamin C in the processing of peas. *Br. Med. Bull.*, **12,** 73

Marcus, M., Prabhudesai, M. and Wassef, S. (1980). Stability of vitamin B_{12} in the presence of ascorbic acid in food and serum: restoration by cyanide of apparent loss. *Am. J. Clin. Nutr.*, **33,** 137

Marks, J. (1968). *The Vitamins in Health and Disease,* p. 131. (London: J. and A. Churchill Ltd.)

Marks, J. (1975). *A Guide to the Vitamins. Their Role in Health and Disease.* (Lancaster, England: MTP Press)

Markwell, N.W. (1947). Vitamin C in the prevention of colds. *Med. J. Aust.*, **2(26),** 777

Marston, H.R. and Dawbarn, M.C. (1941). *Food Composition Tables* (Melbourne: Council for Scientific and Industrial Research), No.107

McClean, H.E., Dodds, P.M., Abernethy, M.H., Stewart, A.W. and Beaven, D.W. (1976). Vitamin C concentration in plasma and leucocytes of men related to age and smoking habit. *NZ Med. J.*, **83(561),** 226

Merigan, T.C. (1974). Quoted by S. Lewin (1974a).

Miller, B.F. and Keane, C.B. (1972). *Encyclopedia and Dictionary of Medicine and Nursing.* (Philadelphia, London, Toronto: W.B. Saunders Co.)

Miller, J.Z., Nance, W.E., Norton, J.A., Wolen, R.L., Griffith, R.S. and Rose, R.J. (1977). Therapeutic effect of vitamin C. A co-twin control study. *J. Am. Med. Assoc.*, **237(3),** 248

Mirvish, S.S. (1975). Blocking the formation of N-nitroso compounds with ascorbic acid *in vitro* and *in vivo*. *Ann. NY Acad. Sci.*, **258,** 175

Moffat, A.C., Patterson, D.A., Currey, A.S. and Owen, P. (1972). Inhibition *in vitro* of cyclic 3′,5′-nucleotide phosphodiesterase activity by drugs. *Europ. J. Toxicol.*, **5(3),** 160

Mohanram, M. and Srikantia, S.G. (1967). Leucocytes and ascorbic acid uptake. *Clin. Sci.*, **32,** 215

Müeller, H.K. and Buschke, W. (1934). *Arch. Augenh.*, **108,** 592. In Wohl, M.G. and Goodhart, R.S. (1970). *Modern Nutrition in Health and Disease,* p. 1033. (Philadelphia: Lea and Febiger)

National Health and Medical Research Council (1971). *Dietary Allowances for Use in Australia.* (Canberra: Australian Government Publishing Service)

National Research Council/Food and Nutrition Board (1948). *Recommended Dietary Allowances*. (Reprint and Circular Series), No 129. (Washington, DC: National Academy of Sciences)

National Research Council/Food and Nutrition Board (1958). *Recommended Dietary Allowances*. Publication 589. (Washington, DC: National Academy of Sciences)

National Research Council/Food and Nutrition Board (1964). *Recommended Dietary Allowances. 6th revised edition*. Publication 1146. (Washington, DC: National Academy of Sciences)

National Research Council/Food and Nutrition Board (1968). *Recommended Dietary Allowances. 7th revised edition*. Publication 1694. (Washington, DC: National Academy of Sciences)

National Research Council/Food and Nutrition Board (1974). *Recommended Dietary Allowances. 8th revised edition*. (Washington, DC: National Academy of Sciences)

National Research Council/Food and Nutrition Board (1980). *Recommended Dietary Allowances. 9th revised edition*. (Washington, DC: National Academy of Sciences)

Newmark, H.L. and Mergens, W.J. (1981). Applications of ascorbic acid and tocopherol as inhibitiors of nitrosamine formation and oxidation in foods. In J. Solms and R.I. Hall (eds.), *Criteria of Food Acceptance*. (Zürich: Forster Verlag)

Nobile, S. (1974a). The nomenclature of vitamins. *Food Technol. Aust.*, **26(4),** 145

Nobile, S. (1974b). Blood vitamin levels in Aboriginal children and their mothers in Western New South Wales. *Med. J. Aust.*, **1,** 601

Nobile, S. (1979). Laboratory investigation of vitamin status. In B.S.Hetzel and S.Nobile, (eds.) *Human Nutrition in Australia*. Suppl. No. 17 to *Int. J. Vit. Nutr. Res.*

Nobile, S. and Woodhill, J.M. (1973). A survey of the vitamin content of some 2000 foods as they are consumed by selected groups of the Australian population. *Food Technol. Aust.*, **25(2),** 80

Nobile, S., Woodhill, J.M. and Rosevear, P.E. (1975). A survey of the vitamin content of foods as they are consumed by selected groups of the Australian population. *Food Technol. Aust.*, **27(9),** 342

Nobile, S., Woodhill, J.M. and Rosevear, P.E. (1976). A survey of the vitamin content of foods as they are consumed by selected groups of the Australian population. *Food Technol. Aust.*, **28(11),** 427

Paul, A.A. and Southgate, D.A.T. (1978). *McCance and Widdowson's The Composition of Foods. 4th revised edition*, Medical Research Council Special Report No. 297 (London: HMSO)

Pauling, L. (1970). *Vitamin C and the Common Cold*. (San Francisco: W.H. Freeman and Company)

Pauling, L. (1979). The role of vitamin C in cancer, In A. Hanck and G. Ritzel (eds.), *Vitamin C*. Suppl. 19 to *Int. J. Vit. Nutr. Res.* pp. 207–210 (Bern: Hans Hubert Verlag)

Pelletier, O. (1968). Smoking and vitamin C levels in humans. *Am. J. Clin. Nutr.*, **21,** 1259

Pelletier, O. (1970). Vitamin C status of cigarette smokers and nonsmokers. *Am. J. Clin. Nutr.*, **23,** 520

Pelletier, O. (1975). Vitamin C and cigarettes smokers. *Ann. NY Acad. Sci.*, **258,** 156

Peterkofsky, B. and Udenfriend, S. (1965). Enzymatic hydroxylation of proline in microsomal polypeptide leading to formation of collagen. *Proc. Nat. Acad. Sci.*,

53, 335
Pitt, H.A. and Costrini, A.M. (1979), Vitamin C prophylaxis in marine recruits. *J. Am. Med. Assoc.*, **241(9),** 908
Plaut, F. and Bülow, M. (1935). Über Unterschiede im C-Vitamingehalt verschiedener Teile des Nerven-systems. *Z. Ges. Neurol. Psychiat.*, **153,** 182
Pure Food Act of New South Wales (1977), *New South Wales Pure Food Act and Regulations* (1977), No. 301, 1908. VCN Blight (Sydney: Government Printer)
Raineri, R. and Weisburger, J.H. (1975). Reduction of gastric carcinogens with ascorbic acid. *Ann. NY Acad. Sci.*, **258,** 181
Randoin, L., Le Gallic, P., Dupuis, Y. and Bernardin, A. (1972). In Jacques Lanore (ed.), *Tables des Composition des Aliments.* (Paris: Institut Scientifique d'Hygiène Alimentaire)
Regnier, E. (1968). The administration of large doses of ascorbic acid in the prevention and treatment of the common cold, Part I and II. *Rev. Allergy*, **22,** 835, 948
Reichstein, T. and Grüssner, A. (1934). *Helv. Chim. Acta*, **17,** 311. In W.H. Sebrell Jr. and R.S. Harris (1967). *The Vitamins, 2nd. Edition, Vol. 1.* (New York: Academic Press Inc.)
Ritzel, G. (1961). Kritische Beurteilung des Vitamins C als Prophylacticum und Therapeuticum der Erkältungskrankheiten. *Helv. Med. Acta*, **28,** 63
Ritzel, G. (1974). Die Beeinflussung der Nährstoffversorgung durch äussere und innere Faktoren, aufgezeigt am Beispiel der Vitamine C and B_1. Suppl. 14 to *Int. J. Vit. Nutr. Res.* G. Brubacher and G. Ritzel (eds.), pp. 80–92 (Bern: Hans Huber Verlag)
Rivers, J.M. (1975). Oral contraceptives and ascorbic acid. *Am. J. Clin. Nutr.*, **28(5),** 550
Rosenberg, H.R. (1945). *Chemistry and Physiology of the Vitamins.* (New York: Interscience Publishers, Inc.)
Sauberlich, H.E. (1975). Vitamin metabolism and requirements: some aspects reviewed. *S.A. Medical J.*, **49,** 2235
Sauberlich, H.E., Dowdy, R.P. and Skala, J.H. (1974). *Laboratory Tests for the Assessment of Nutritional Status.* (Cleveland, Ohio: CRC Press Inc.)
Schaus, R. (1957). The ascorbic acid content of human pituitary, cerebral cortex, heart and skeletal muscle and its relation to age. *Am. J. Clin. Nutr.*, **5,** 39
Scheinberg, I.H. (1966). Biochemistry of copper. In M.G. Wohl and R.S. Goodhart (1970) *Modern Nutrition in Health and Disease*, p. 383. (Philadelphia: Lea and Febiger)
Schneider, W. and Staudinger, H. (1965). Reduced nictotinamide-adenine dinucleotide dependent reduction of semidehydroascorbic acid. *Biochim. Biophys. Acta*, **96,** 157
Schrauzer, C.N. and Rhead, W.J. (1973). Ascorbic acid abuse: effects of longterm ingestion of excessive amounts on blood levels and urinary excretion. *Int. J. Vit. Nutr. Res.*, **43,** 201
Schwartz, A.B., Togo, Y., Hornick, R.B., Tominaga, S. and Gleckman, R.A. (1973). Evaluation of the efficacy of ascorbic acid in prophylaxis of induced rhinovirus 44 infection in man. *J. Infect. Dis.*, **128,** 500
Sebrell, W.H. Jr. and Harris, R.S. (1967). *The Vitamins, Chemistry, Physiology, Pathology, Methods. 2nd. Edition, Vol. 1.* (New York: Academic Press Inc.)
Sherman, H.C. (1946). *Chemistry of Food and Nutrition, 7th edition.* (New York: The Macmillan Company)
Siest, G., Appel, W., Blijenberg, G.B., Capolaghi, B., Galteau, M.M., Heusghem, C., Hjelm, M., Lauer, K.L., Le Perron, B., Loppinet, V., Love, C.,

Royer, R.J., Tognoni, C. and Wilding P. (1978). Drug interference in clinical chemistry: studies on ascorbic acid. *J. Clin. Chem. Clin. Biochem.*, **16(2),** 103
Sigurjonsson, J. (1951). Excretion of vitamin C in urine following repeated administration of big test doses. *Br. J. Nutr.*, **5,** 216
Silink, S.J., Nobile, S. and Woodhill, J.M. (1972). Clinical and biochemical asessment of nutritional status. *J. Geriatr.*, **October 27.** Reprinted in *Mod. Geriatr.*, **July/August** (1973)
Spencer, R.P., Purdy, S., Hoeldtke, R., Bow, T.M. and Markulis, M.A. (1963). Studies on intestinal absorption of L-ascorbic acid 1–^{14}C. *Gastroenterology*, **44,** 768
Spittle, C.R. (1973). Atherosclerosis and vitamin C. *Lancet*, **2,** 199
Stein, H.B., Hasan, A. and Fox, I.H. (1976). Ascorbic acid-induced uricosuria. A consequence of megavitamin therapy. *Ann. Intern. Med.*, **84(4),** 385
Street, J.C. and Chadwick, R.W. (1975). Ascorbic acid requirements and metabolism in relation to organochlorine pesticides. *Ann. NY Acad. Sci.*, **258,** 132
Stucky, V. (1979). *Nutrition for the Nation: Points Simplified.* (Overland Park, Kansas: Nutrition Education Centre)
Szent-Györgyi, A. (1928). *Biochem. J.*, **22,** 1387. In W.H. Sebrell Jr. and R.S. Harris (1967). *The Vitamins, 2nd Edition, Vol. 1.* (New York: Academic Press Inc.)
Szent-Györgyi, A. (1979). How vitamin C really works ... or does it? *Nutr. Today*, **September/October,** 6, 15
Szent-Györgyi, A. and Haworth, W.N. (1933). *Nature*, **131,** 23. In W.H. Sebrell Jr. and R.S. Harris (1967). *The Vitamins, 2nd Edition, Vol. 1.* (New York: Academic Press. Inc.)
Tebrock, H.E., Arminio, J.J. and Johnston, J.H. (1956). Usefulness of bioflavonoids and ascorbic acid in treatment of common cold. *J. Am. Med. Assoc.*, **162,** 1227
Terroine, T. (1960). The vitamins interrelations of ascorbic acid. *World Rev. Nutr. Diet.*, **2,** 105
Terroine, T. (1966). *Les Interrelations Vitaminiques.* (Paris: Ed. Centre National de la Recherche Scientifique)
Thomas, S. and Corden, M. (1970; 1977). *Tables of Composition of Australian Foods* (Canberra: Australian Government Publishing Service)
Tillmans, J. (1930) *Z. Untersuch. Lebensm*, **60,** 34. In W.H. Sebrell Jr., and R.S. Harris (1967). *The Vitamins, 2nd Edition, Vol. 1.* (New York: Academic Press Inc.)
Tisdale, M.J. (1975). Inhibition of cyclic adenosine 3′,5′–monophosphate phosphodiesterase from Walker carcinoma by ascorbic acid and dehydroascorbic acid. *Biochem. Biophys. Res. Commun.*, **61,** 877
Todhunter, E.N. and Robbins, R.C. (1940). Observations on the amount of ascorbic acid required to maintain tissue saturation in normal adults. *J. Nutr.*, **19,** 263
Tyrrell, D.A.J. (1965). *Common Colds and Related Disease.* (London: Edward Arnold Ltd.)
Tyrrell, D.A., Craig, J.W., Meada, T.W. and White, T. (1977). A trial of ascorbic acid in the treatment of the common cold. *Br. J. Prev. Soc. Med.*, **31(3),** 189
Vilter, R.W. (1967). Ascorbic acid requirements of man. In W.H. Sebrell Jr. and R.S.Harris, *The Vitamins, 2nd. Edition, Vol. 1.* (New York: Academic Press Inc.)
Vilter, R.W. (1970). Vitamin C (ascorbic acid). In M.G.Wohl and R.S. Goodhart, *Modern Nutrition in Health and Disease,* pp. 296–312. (Philadelphia: Lea and Febiger)
Vuillemier, J.P. (1967). Analytische Probleme bei der Bestimmung von Vitamin C

im Zusammenhang mit Ernährungserhebungen. *Int. Z. Vitaminforsch.*, **37,** 504
Wagner, A.F. and Folkers, K.A. (1964). *Vitamins and Coenzymes.* p. 208. (New York: Interscience Publishers Inc.)
Walker, G.H., Bynoe, M.L. and Tyrrell, D.A.J. (1967). Trial of ascorbic acid in prevention of colds. *Br. Med. J.*, **1,** 603
Watt, B.K. and Merrill A.L. (1963). *Composition of Foods, Raw, Processed, Prepared. Agriculture Handbook No. 8.* (Washington, DC: Agricultural Service, US Department of Agriculture)
Waugh, W.A. and King, C.G. (1932). *J. Biol. Chem.*, **97,** 325. In W.H. Sebrell Jr. and R.S.Harris (1967). *The Vitamins, 2nd. Edition, Vol. 1.* (New York: Academic Press Inc.)
Weis, W. (1975). Ascorbic acid and electron transport. *Ann. NY Acad. Sci.*, **258,** 190
Williams, R.C., Baker, D.R. and Schmit, J.A. (1973). Analysis of water soluble vitamins by high-speed ion-exchange chromatography. *J. Chromat. Sci.*, **11,** 618
Willis, G.C., Light, A.W. and Gow, W.S. (1954). *Can. Med. Assoc. J.*, **71,** 526
Wilson, C.W.M. (1971). Vitamin C and the common cold. Letter to the Editor. *Br. Med. J.*, **1(5750),** 669
Wilson, C.W.M. (1973a). *Vitamine*, **iii,** 75. (Basle: Ed. Roche)
Wilson, C.W.M. (1973b). The transfer and utilisation of vitamin C as interpreted by its human biological rhythms. In Scheving, Halberg, and Pauly (eds.), *Chronobiology, Proceedings, Congress of the International Society for the Study of Biological Rhythms*, pp. 249–255. (Little Rock, Ark.). (Tokyo: Igaku Shoin)
Wilson, C. (1973c). Vitamin C makes colds less complex. *New Sci.*, **29 March,** 712
Wilson, C.W.M. (1973d). Ascorbic acid and the common cold. *Br. Med. J.*, **IV,** 166
Wilson, C.W.M. (1974). Vitamin C. Tissue saturation, metabolism and desaturation. *Practitioner*, **212,** 481
Wilson, C.W.M. (1975a). Colds, ascorbic acid metabolism, and vitamin C. *J.Clin. Pharmacol.*, **15(8–9),** 570
Wilson, C.W.M. (1975b). Clinical pharmacological aspects of ascorbic acid. *Ann. NY Acad. Sci.*, **258,** 355
Wilson, C.W.M. (1975c). Ascorbic acid function and metabolism during colds. *Ann. NY Acad. Sci.*, **258,** 529
Wilson, C.W.M. (1975d). Colds and vitamin C. *Irish Med. J.*, **68(20),** 511
Wilson, C.W.M. (1975e). Ascorbic acid and the common cold. *Practitioner*, **215(1287),** 343
Wilson, C.W.M. (1976a). Vitamin C and the common cold. Letter to the Editor. *Br. Med. J.*, **1(6023),** 1470
Wilson, C.W.M. (1976b). Vitamin C for common colds. Letter to the Editor. *Lancet*, **1(7959),** 586
Wilson, C.W.M. and Greene, M. (1978). The relationship of aspirin to ascorbic acid metabolism during the common cold. *J. Clin. Pharmacol.*, **18(1),** 21
Wilson, C.W.M., Greene, M. and Loh, H.S. (1976). The metabolism of supplementary vitamin C during the common cold. *J. Clin. Pharmacol.*, **16(1),** 19
Wilson, C.W.M. and Loh, H.S. (1969a). Studies in ascorbic acid taste threshold circadian rhythm in relation to plasma ascorbic acid levels. *Irish J. Med. Sci.*, **2,** 396
Wilson, C.W.M. and Loh, H.S. (1969b). Ascorbic acid and upper respiratory inflammation. *Acta Allergol.*, **XXIV,** 367
Wilson, C.W.M. and Loh, H.S. (1973). Common cold and vitamin C. *Lancet*, **1,** 638
Wilson, C.W.M., Loh, H.S. and Foster, F.G. (1973a). The beneficial effect of

vitamin C on the common cold. *Europ. J. Clin. Pharmacol.*, **6,** 26
Wilson, C.W.M., Loh, H.S. and Foster, F.G. (1973b). Common cold symptomatology and vitamin C. *Europ. J. Clin. Pharmacol.*, **6,** 196
Wohl, M.G. and Goodhart, R.S. (1970). *Modern Nutrition in Health and Disease.* (Phildelphia: Lea and Febiger), p. 324
Wolbach, S.B. (1937). The pathological changes resulting from vitamin deficiency. *J. Am. Med. Assoc.*, **108,** 7
Woodhill, J.M. (1951). The influence of maternal diet upon the course and outcome of pregnancy in a group of Australian women. A thesis submitted to the Faculty of The Harvard School of Public Health in Partial Fulfillment of the Requirements for the Degree of Doctor of Science in Hygiene. (Boston, Massachusetts)
Woodhill, J.M. (1970). Australian dietary surveys with special reference to vitamins. *Int. J. Vit. Res.*, **40(4),** 520
Woodhill, J.M. (1979). Assessment of diet. In B.S.Hetzel and S. Nobile (eds.) *Human Nutrition in Australia.* Suppl. No. 17 to *Int. J. Vit. Nutr. Res.*
Woodhill, J.M. and Nobile, S. (1971a). Vitamin C (L-ascorbic acid and dehydro-L-ascorbic acid). A contribution to the Captain Cook bicentennial celebrations. *Med. Aust.*, **1,** 1009
Woodhill, J.M. and Nobile, S. (1971b). Ascorbic acid. *Am. J. Clin. Nutr.*, **24(11),** 1301 (Letter)
Woodhill, J.M. and Nobile, S. (1972). Nutrition in the elderly – calories, protein and vitamin C. *J. Geriatr.*, **3,** 35. Reprinted in *Mod. Geriatr,* **July/August** (1973)
Woodhill, J.M., Nobile, S., Silink, S.J. and Winston, J.M. (1974). Case studies on the nutritional status of socially deprived children in Sydney. *Aust. Paediatr. J.*, **10,** 199
World Health Organisation (1963). Technical Report Series No. 258. Expert committee on medical assessment of nutritional status. Geneva.
Yamazaki, I., Mason, H.S. and Piette, L. (1959). Identification of intermediate substrate free-radicals formed during peroxidatic oxidations, by electron paramagnetic resonance spectroscopy. *Biochem. Biophys. Res. Comm.*, **1(6),** 336
Yamazaki, I., Mason, H.S. and Piette, L. (1960). Identification, by electron paramagnetic resonance spectroscopy, of free radicals generated from substrates by peroxidase. *J. Biol. Chem.*, **235,** 2444
Yamazaki, I. and Piette, L.H. (1961). Mechanism of free radical formation and disappearance during the ascorbic acid oxidase and peroxidase reactions. *Biochem. Biophys. Acta*, **50,** 62
Yavorsky, M., Almaden, P. and King, C.G. (1934). The vitamin C content of human tissues. *J. Biol. Chem.*, **106,** 525
Zilva, S.S. (1923). *Biochem. J.* **17,** 410 and 416. In W.H. Sebrell Jr. and R.S. Harris (1967). *The Vitamins, 2nd. Edition, Vol. 1.* (New York: Academic Press Inc.)
Zilva, S.S. (1927). *Biochem. J.*, **21,** 689. In W.H. Sebrell Jr. and R.S. Harris (1967). *The Vitamins, 2nd. Edition, Vol. 1.*(New York: Academic Press Inc.)

15.1 SPECIAL REFERENCES TO VITAMIN C AND THE COMMON COLD

Adams, R. and Murray, F. (1972). *Vitamin C, the Powerhouse Vitamin – Conquers More than Just Colds.* (New York: Larchmont Press)
Anderson, T.W. (1975). Large-scale trials of vitamin C. *Ann. NY Acad. Sci.*, **258,** 498

Anderson, T.W. (1977). Large scale studies with vitamin C. *Acta Vitaminol. Enzymol.* (Milano), **31(1–5),** 43
Anderson, T.W. (1979). Vitamin C: cure for the common cold? *Am. Pharm.*, **19(2),** 46
Anderson, T.W., Reid, D.B.W. and Beaton, G.H. (1972). Vitamin C and the common cold. A double-blind trial. *Can. Med. Assoc. J.*, **107,** 503
Anderson, T.W., Suranyi, G. and Beaton, G.H. (1974). The effect on winter illness of large doses of vitamin C. *Can. Med. Assoc. J.*, **111,** 31
Anderson, T.W., Beaton, G.H., Corey, P. and Spero, L. (1975). Winter illness and vitamin C: the effect of relatively low doses. *Can. Med. Assoc. J.*, **112(7),** 823
Baird, I.M., Hughes, R.E., Wilson, H.K., Davies, J.E.W. and Howard, A.N. (1979). The effects of ascorbic acid and flavonoids on the occurrence of symptoms normally associated with the common cold. *Am. J. Clin. Nutr.*, **32(8),** 1686
Banks, H.S. (1968). Controlled trials in the early antibiotic treatment of colds. *Med. Officer,* **119,** 7
Barnes, F.E. (1961). Vitamin C supplements and the incidence of colds in High School basketball players. *N. Carolina Med. J.*, **22,** 22
British Medical Journal – Editorial (1973). Ascorbic acid and common colds. *Br. Med. J.*, **3(5875),** 311
British Medical Journal – Editorial (1976). Vitamin C and the common cold. *Br. Med. J.*, **1(6010),** 606
Broadhurst, N.A. and Crafter, K.C. (1975). Vitamin C and the common cold. *Austr. Family Physician,* **4 (April),** 271, 275, 277.
Caels, F. (1953). Contribution a l'etude de l'effet de hautes doses de vitamine C dans les infections oto-rhino-laryngologiques. *Acta Oto-Rhino-Laryngol. Belg.*, **7,** 395
Chalmers, T.C. (1974). Quoted by S. Lewin (1974a)
Chalmers, T.C. (1975). Effects of ascorbic acid on the common cold. An evaluation of the evidence. *Am. J. Med.*, **58(4),** 532
Charleston, S.S. and Clegg, K.M. (1972). Ascorbic acid and the common cold. *Lancet,* **1,** 1401
Cheraskin, E., Ringsdorf, W.M., Michael, D.W. and Hicks, B.S. (1973). Daily vitamin C consumption and reported respiratory findings. *Int. J. Vit. Nutr. Res.*, **43,** 42
Clegg, K.M. and MacDonald, J.M. (1975a). L-ascorbic acid and D-isoascorbic acid in a common cold survey. *Am. J. Clin. Nutr.*, **28(9),** 973
Clegg, K.M. and MacDonald, J.M. (1975b). D-isoascorbic acid investigated in a common cold survey. *Proc. Nutr. Soc.*, **34(1),** 7A
Colby, R.H., Brown, J., Fine, R. and Karlson, R. (1974). Quoted by S. Lewin (1974a)
Cook, J.D. and Monsen, E.R. (1977). Vitamin C, the common cold, and iron absorption. *Am. J. Clin. Nutr.*, **30(2),** 235
Coulehan, J.L. (1979). Ascorbic acid and the common cold: reviewing the evidence. *Postgrad. Med.*, **66(3),** 153, 157, 160
Coulehan, J.L., Reisinger, K.S., Rogers, K.D. and Bradley, D.W. (1974). Vitamin C prophylaxis in a boarding school. *N. Engl. J. Med.*, **290,** 6
Coulehan, J.L., Kapner, L., Eberhard, S., Taylor, F.H. and Rogers, K.D. (1975). Vitamin C and upper respiratory illness in Navaho children: preliminary observations (1974). *Ann. NY Acad. Sci.*, **258,** 513
Coulehan, J.L., Eberhard, S., Kapner, L., Taylor, F., Rogers, K. and Garry, P. (1976). Vitamin C and acute illness in Navaho school children. *N. Engl. J. Med.*, **295(18),** 973

Cowan, D.W., Diehl, H.S. and Baker, A.B. (1942). Vitamins for the prevention of colds. Maximum dose of 500 mg vitamin C. *J. Am. Med. Assoc.*, **120,** 1267

Dahlberg, G., Engel, A. and Rydin, H. (1944). The value of ascorbic acid as a prophylactic against 'common colds'. *Acta Med. Scand.*, **119,** 540

Dietz, N. Jr, (1957). The common cold and stress conditions. *Indust. Med. Surg.*, **26(5),** 229

Drug and Therapeutic Information Inc., New York. (1970). Vitamin C and the common cold. *The Medical Letter*, **12(26),** 105

Dykes, M.H.M. and Meier, P. (1975). Ascorbic acid and the common cold. Evaluation of its efficacy and toxicity. *J. Am. Med. Assoc.*, **231(10),** 1073

Elwood, P.C., Lee, H.P., St. Leger, A.S., Baird, M. and Howard, A.N. (1976). A randomized controlled trial of vitamin C in the prevention and amelioration of the common cold. *Br. J. Prev. Soc. Med.*, **30(3),** 193

Elwood, P.C., Hughes, S.J. and Leger, A.S. (1977). A randomized controlled trial of the therapeutic effect of vitamin C in the common cold. *Practitioner*, **218(1303),** 133

Franz, W.L., Sands, G.W. and Heyl, H.L. (1956). Blood ascorbic acid level in bioflavonoid and ascorbic acid therapy of common cold. *J. Am. Med. Assoc.*, **162,** 1224

General Practitioner Trials (1968). Ineffectiveness of vitamin C in treating coryza. *Practitioner*, **200,** 442

Glazebrook, A.J. and Thomson, S. (1942). The administration of vitamin C in a large institution and its effect on general health and resistance to infection. *J. Hyg.*, **42(1),** 1

Greene, M. and Wilson, C.W. (1975). Effect of aspirin on ascorbic acid metabolism during colds (proceedings). *Br. J. Clin. Pharmacol.*, **2(4),** 369P

Hume, R. and Weyers, E. (1973). Changes in leucocyte ascorbic acid during the common cold. *Scot. Med. J.*, **18,** 3

Karlowski, T.R., Chalmers, T.C., Frenkel, L.D., Kapikian, A.Z., Lewis, T.L. and Lynch, J.M. (1975). Ascorbic acid for the common cold. A prophylactic and therapeutic trial. *J. Am. Med. Assoc.*, **231(10),** 1038

Kent, S. (1978). Vitamin C therapy: colds, cancer, and cardiovascular disease. *Geriatrics*, **33(10),** 91

Lewin, S. (1974a). Vitamin C and the common cold. Abbreviated report of the 1973 international conference held in Stanford. *Chem. Br.*, **10(1),** 25

Lewin, S. (1974b). The use of megaquantities of ascorbic acid or ascorbate for therapeutic and prophylactic purposes in relation to biochemical individuality. *Biochem. Soc. Trans.*, **2,** 154

Lewin, S. (1974c). The ascorbate system and the formation of adenosine 3':5'-cyclic monophosphate. *Biochem. Soc. Trans.*, **2,** 400

Lewin, S. (1976). *Vitamin C: Its Molecular Biology and Medical Potential.* (London, New York: Academic Press)

Lewis, T.L., Karlowski, T.R., Kapikian, A.Z., Lynch, J.M., Shaffer, G.W., George, D.A. and Chalmers, T.C. (1975). A controlled clinical trial of ascorbic acid for the common cold. *Ann. NY Acad. Sci.*, **258,** 505

Loh, H.S. and Wilson, C.W.M. (1970). The origin of ascorbic acid stored in the leucocytes. *Br. J. Pharmacol.*, **40,** 169P

Loh, H.S. and Wilson, C.W.M. (1971a). An improved method for the measurement of leucocyte ascorbic acid concentrations. *Int. J. Vit. Nutr. Res.*, **41,** 90

Loh, H.S. and Wilson, C.W.M. (1971b). Relationship between leucocyte and plasma ascorbic acid concentrations. *Br. Med. J.*, **3,** 733

Loh, H.S. and Wilson, C.W.M. (1971c). The relationship between leucocyte ascorbic acid and haemoglobin levels at different ages. *Int. J. Vit. Nutr. Res.*, **41,** 259

Loh, H.S. and Wilson, C.W.M. (1971d). The relationship between leucocyte ascorbic acid concentrations and the total white blood count. *Int. J. Vit. Nutr. Res.*, **41,** 253

Ludvigsson, J., Hansson, L.O. and Tibbling, G. (1977). Vitamin C as a preventive medicine against common colds in children. *Scand. J. Infect. Dis.*, **9(2),** 91

Marks, J. (1975). *A Guide to the Vitamins. Their Role in Health and Disease.* (Lancaster, England: MTP Press)

Markwell, N.W. (1947). Vitamin C in the prevention of colds. *Med. J. Aust.*, **2(26),** 777

Merigan, T.C. (1974). Quoted by S.Lewin (1974a).

Miller, B.F. and Keane, C.B. (1972). *Encyclopedia and Dictionary of Medicine and Nursing*. (Philadelphia, London, Toronto: W.B. Saunders Co.)

Miller, J.Z., Nance, W.E., Norton, J.A., Wolen, R.L., Griffith, R.S. and Rose, R.J. (1977). Therapeutic effect of vitamin C. A co-twin control study. *J. Am. Med. Assoc.*, **237(3),** 248

Moffat, A.C., Patterson, D.A., Currey, A.S. and Owen, P. (1972). Inhibition *in vitro* of cyclic 3′,5′ nucleotide phosophodiesterase activity by drugs. *Europ. J. Toxicol.*, **5(3),** 160

Nitsche, W. (1973). Vitamin C and its indications. *Med. Monatsschr.*, **27(10),** 454

Nutrition Reviews – Editorial (1967). Ascorbic acid and the common cold. *Nutr. Rev.*, **25(8),** 228

Pauling, L. (1970). *Vitamin C and the Common Cold.* (San Francisco: W.H. Freeman and Co.)

Pauling, L. (1971a). The significance of the evidence about ascorbic acid and the common cold. *Proc. Natl. Acad. Sci. USA*, **68,** 2678

Pauling, L. (1971b). Ascorbic acid and the common cold. *Am. J. Clin. Nutr.*, **24,** 1294

Pauling, L.C. (1976). *Vitamin C, the Common Cold and the Flu.* (San Francisco: W.H. Freeman and Co.)

Pitt, H.A. and Costrini, A.M. (1979). Vitamin C prophylaxis in marine recruits. *J. Am. Med. Assoc.*, **241(9),** 908

Preshaw, R.M. (1972). Vitamin C and the common cold. Editorials. *Can. Med. Assoc. J.*, **107,** 479

Regnier, E. (1968). The administration of large doses of ascorbic acid in the prevention and treatment of the common cold, Part I and II. *Rev. Allergy,* **22,** 835, 948

Ritzel, G. (1961). Kritische Beurteilung des Vitamins C als Prophylacticum und Therapeuticum der Erkältungskrankheiten. *Helv. Med. Acta,* **28,** 63

Ritzel, G. (1976). Ascorbic acid and the common cold. Letter to the Editor. *J. Am. Med. Assoc.*, **235 (11),** 1108

Schwartz, A.R., Togo, Y., Hornick, R.B., Tominaga, S. and Gleckman, R.A. (1973). Evaluation of the efficacy of ascorbic acid in prophylaxis of induced rhinovirus 44 infection in man. *J. Infect. Dis.*, **128,** 500

Spero, L.M. and Anderson, T.W. (1973). Ascorbic acid and the common cold. Letter to the Editor. *Br. Med. J.*, **4,** 354

Stone, I. (1972). *The Healing Factor: Vitamin C Against Disease.* (New York: Grosset and Dunlap)

Taft, G. and Fieldhouse, P. (1978). Vitamin C and the common cold. *Publ. Health,* **92(1),** 19

Tebrock, H.E., Arminio, J.J. and Johnston, J.H. (1956). Usefulness of bioflavonoids and ascorbic acid in treatment of common cold. *J. Am. Med. Assoc.*, **162,** 1227

Tisdale, M.J. (1975). Inhibition of cyclic adenosine 3′,5′-monophosphate phosphodiesterase from Walker carcinoma by ascorbic acid and dehydroascorbic acid. *Biochem. Biophys. Res. Commun.*, **61,** 877

Tyrrell, D.A.J. (1965). *Common Colds and Related Diseases.* (London: Edward Arnold Ltd.)

Tyrrell, D.A., Craig, J.W., Meada, T.W. and White, T. (1977). A trial of ascorbic acid in the treatment of the common cold. *Br. J. Prev. Soc. Med.*, **31(3),** 189

Walker, G.H., Bynoe, M.L. and Tyrrell, D.A.J. (1967). Trial of ascorbic acid in prevention of colds. *Br. Med. J.*, **1,** 603

Wilson, C.W.M. (1971). Vitamin C and the common cold. Letter to the Editor. *Br. Med. J.*, **1(5750),** 669

Wilson, C.W.M. (1973c). Vitamin C makes cold less complex. *New Sci.*, **29 March,** 712

Wilson, C.W.M. (1973d). Ascorbic acid and the common cold. *Br. Med. J.*, **IV,** 166

Wilson, C.W.M. (1974). Vitamin C.Tissue saturation, metabolism and desaturation. *Practitioner*, **212,** 481

Wilson, C.W.M. (1975a). Colds, ascorbic acid metabolism, and vitamin C. *J. Clin. Pharmacol.*, **15(8–9),** 570

Wilson, C.W.M. (1975b). Clinical pharmacological aspects of ascorbic acid. *Ann. NY Acad. Sci.*, **258,** 355

Wilson, C.W.M. (1975c). Ascorbic acid function and metabolism during colds. *Ann. NY Acad. Sci.*, **258,** 529

Wilson, C.W.M. (1975d). Colds and vitamin C. *Irish Med. J.*, **68(20),** 511

Wilson, C.W.M. (1975e). Ascorbic acid and the common cold. *Practitioner*, **215(1287),** 343

Wilson, C.W.M. (1976a). Vitamin C and the common cold. Letter to the Editor. *Br. Med. J.*, **1(6023),** 1470

Wilson, C.W.M. (1976b). Vitamin C for common colds. Letter to the Editor. *Lancet*, **1(7959),** 586

Wilson, C.W.M. and Greene, M. (1978). The relationship of aspirin to ascorbic acid metabolism during the common cold. *J. Clin. Pharmacol.*, **18(1),** 21

Wilson, C.W.M. and Loh, H.S. (1969b). Ascorbic acid and upper respiratory inflammation. *Acta Allergol.*, **XXIV,** 367

Wilson, C.W.M. and Loh, H.S. (1973). Common cold and vitamin C. *Lancet*, **1,** 638

Wilson, C.W.M., Loh, H.S. and Foster, F.G. (1973a). The beneficial effect of vitamin C on the common cold. *Europ. J. Clin. Pharmacol.*, **6,** 26

Wilson, C.W.M., Loh, H.S. and Foster, F.G., (1973b). Common cold symptomatology and vitamin C. *Europ. J. Clin. Pharmacol.*, **6,** 196

Wilson, C.W.M., Greene, M., and Loh, H.S. (1976). The metabolism of supplementary vitamin C during the common cold. *J. Clin. Pharmacol.*, **161(1),** 19

16
Abbreviations, symbols and glossary

16.1 ABBREVIATIONS

AA =	L-ascorbic acid
ACTH =	adrenocorticotropic hormone, corticotropin
cAMP =	cyclic adenosine 3′, 5′-monophosphate
ATP =	adenosine triphosphate
CSIR =	Council for Scientific Industrial Research, Australia (now CSIRO)
DHAA =	dehydro-L-ascorbic acid
DNA =	deoxyribonucleic acid
FAO =	Food and Agricultural Organization, Rome
FAD =	flavin adenine dinucleotide
FNB –	Food and Nutrition Board of the NRC, USA
cGMP =	cyclic guanosine 3′,5′-monophosphate
HPLC =	high pressure liquid chromatography
ICNND =	Interdepartmental Committee on Nutrition for National Defense
IR =	infrared
MDHAA =	monodehydro-L-ascorbic acid
NAD =	nicotinamide adenine dinucleotide
NADH =	nicotinamide adenine dinucleotide, reduced
NH and MRC =	National Health and Medical Research Council, Australia
NRC =	National Research Council, United States
n.s. =	not significant (statistically)
PALP =	pyridoxal-5′-phosphate
ProA =	provitamin A = beta-carotene
RNA =	ribonucleic acid
SD =	standard deviation – statistics
t.d.s. =	three times daily
TPP =	thiamine pyrophosphate
UV =	ultraviolet
WHO =	World Health Organization, Geneva

16.2 SYMBOLS

α =	alpha (Greek letter) used in chemical formulae
$[\alpha]_D^{20^\circ}$	indicates the specific optical rotation of a substance at 20 °C for D-line of sodium light
β =	beta (Greek letter) used in chemical formulae
C =	carbon atom
^{14}C =	radioactive carbon isotope
°C =	degrees centigrade (temperature)
Ca =	calcium
cm =	centimetre = 10^{-2} m
Cu =	copper
D =	*dextro* : rotates polarized light to the right
e =	electron
ε =	epsilon (Greek letter): indicates the intensity of light absorption of 1 g of substance in 100 ml of a particular solvent in a cell having an absorption path of 1 cm
Fe =	iron
g =	gram
γ =	gamma (Greek letter) used in chemical formulae, also to define some radiation (gamma rays) and sometimes to express micrograms (μg)
H =	hydrogen atom
Hg =	mercury
IU =	international unit (eg 1 IU vitamin A = 0.344 μg pure retinyl acetate)
λ =	lambda (Greek letter) : indicates the wavelength
λ_{max} =	wavelength of maximum absorption
L =	*laevo* : rotates polarized light to the left.
mg =	milligram = 10^{-3} g
Mg =	magnesium
μg =	microgram = 10^{-6} g
ml =	millilitre = 10^{-3} l
μl =	microlitre = 10^{-6} l
N =	nitrogen
N =	normal solution (applied to concentrations)
Na =	sodium
ng =	nanogram = 10^{-9} g
NH_4 =	ammonium ion
nm =	nanometre: 10^{-1} nm = 1 Ångström unit
o =	*ortho:* indicates the position of a radical (group) in the benzene ring
O =	oxygen atom
−OH =	hydroxyl group or ion
p =	*para:* indicates the position of a radical (group) in the benzene ring
pH =	acid-base scale; log of reciprocal of hydrogen ion concentration
pK =	dissociation constant
R =	radical or group (e.g. methyl CH_3)
−SH− =	sulphydryl group
−S–S− =	disulphide (two sulphur atoms linked together)

16.3 GLOSSARY

Absorption in physiology: uptake and incorporation of a substance into a body fluid or tissue.

Absorption of light: see **absorption spectrum**

Absorption spectrum: when dispersed light of definite wavelength or frequency ranges (e.g. IR light: 25 000–750 nm; visible light: 750–400 nm; UV light: 400–200 nm) passes through a solution of a particular substance, this absorbs, in a characteristic manner, certain components of the light leaving darkened areas in the transmitted spectrum. This is called the absorption spectrum or absorption curve. It exhibits maxima and minima, the maxima corresponding to the presence in the molecule of the substance of certain groups of atoms called chromophores. The instruments for measuring absorption spectra are called IR, visible or UV-spectrophotometers.

Acrolein: acrylic aldehyde, $CH_2{=}CH{\cdot}CHO$, irritates skin and mucous membranes, formed in cigarette smoke.

Adenosine triphosphate–ATP: a coenzyme acting in the transfer of pyrophosphate bond energy. Hydrolysis of these bonds releases the energy necessary to the living cell to perform various work, such as contraction of muscles, production of secretion, activities of nervous system, and synthesis of cell constituents.

Adrenal gland (s): a small endocrine gland that rests on top of each kidney. Each adrenal gland is a gland within a gland: the outer shell or cortex and the inner core or medulla.

Adrenaline (epinephrine): a hormone produced by the adrenal medulla or inner core of the adrenal glands. It stimulates the heart, increases heart rate and raises blood pressure.

Adrenochromes: toxic oxidation products of adrenaline.

Adsorption in chemistry: concentration or accumulation of, e.g., a liquid on the surface of, e.g., a solid with which it becomes in contact (see **chromatography**).

Aerobic: (e.g. of reaction) requiring free oxygen.

Aliquot: a part of the whole; a sample which represents the whole.

Alkaline phosphatase: enzyme present in most cells, particularly in zones of growth of bones, intestinal mucosa, kidneys, lactating mammary gland, milk. It might serve to provide inorganic phosphate for metabolic, excretory and some secretory purposes.

Amines: organic compounds containing nitrogen bound to a carbon atom. Formulae: R–NH; R–NR; $R{-}NH_2$.

Amino acids: organic acids containing nitrogen. Formula: $R{-}NH_2{\cdot}COOH$. They form the building units of protein.

Aminotransferases: enzymes active in transferring nitrogenous groups.

Anabolism: see **metabolism**.

Anaemia: a condition manifesting in unhealthy paleness and due to deficiency of various nutrients, principally of iron and the vitamins B_c (folic acid) and B_{12}.

Anaerobic: (e.g. of reaction) not requiring free oxygen.

Analgesic: a substance which relieves pain.

Analysis: determination of the elements of a compound (e.g. food, tissue, body fluid). It can be qualitative, i.e. determine the presence of the element(s), or quantitative, i.e. determine the amount of the element(s).

Angular palpebritis: excoriation and fissuring of the external canthi (angles of the eyelids).

Angular stomatitis: sodden and excoriated lesions associated with fissuring at the angles of the mouth.

Anion: negative ion.

Anthropometric: pertaining to measures (metric) of the human body (*anthropos* = man).

Antibody: a protein that is produced in the body in response to invasion by a foreign agent (= **antigen**) that reacts specifically with it.

Anti-coagulant: any substance that inhibits the blood clotting mechanism.

Antigen: see **antibody**.

Anti-histamines: drugs that counteract the effect of histamine, a natural constituent of many tissues and blood, which is innocuous when in a bound or inactive form but injurious when released in a free form into body fluids as a result of certain stimuli.

Anti-inflammatory: working against inflammation, a morbid process affecting some part of the body, characterised by excessive heat, swelling, pain and redness.

Apo-enzyme: the protein moiety of an enzyme (holo-enzyme).

Ascites: abnormal building up of fluid in the peritoneal cavity.

Aspartate: a salt of aspartic acid, a non-essential amino acid occurring in animal and plant tissues.

Asymmetric carbon atom: one containing a different atom or radical on each of its four valence bonds.

Atheroma: a lesion in the walls of the arteries in which cholesterol is deposited.

Atherosclerosis: hardening of the walls of the arteries and sometimes the valves of the heart.

Atrophic: wasted away through improper nourishment.

Auto-oxidation: spontaneous oxidation occurring in very unstable compounds, e.g. when exposed to atmospheric oxygen.

Bacteriophage: a virus that multiplies in bacteria and destroys them.

Bacterium (plural **bacteria**): microscopic unicellular organism.

Benzoates: salts of benzoic acid used in the preservation of foods and as anti-fungal agents.

Beri-beri: a deficiency disease caused by the lack of vitamin B_1. Symptoms are polyneuritis and disturbances of the central nervous system.

Bidistilled: water twice distilled in all-glass containers.

Bilirubin: main pigment of the bile, normally found in blood, increased levels in liver disease.

Biopsy: sample of living material removed for examination purposes by cut or puncture.

Biosynthesis: formation of new compounds within the body.

Bitot's spots: triangular whitish foamy patches developing at the eye corners, thought to be due to a vitamin A deficiency.

Body water: total extracellular water plus cell residue.

Bronchial (adjective of Bronchi) two of the main divisions of the wind-pipe conveying air to the lungs, hence bronchitis.

Bronchitis: inflammation of the bronchi.

Butanol: a lower alcohol, $C_3H_7CH_2OH$.

Calculi: small hard masses formed in pathological conditions chiefly in the hollow organs of the body (e.g. kidneys) or their passages, consisting of salts of acids such as oxalic acid or uric acid; also called stones.

Carbohydrates: sugars (mono and poly-saccharides), carbon compounds containing hydrogen and oxygen in the ratio 2 : 1, general formula: $C_x(H_2O)_y$.

Carbon bonds: linkages between two atoms of carbon, $\rightarrow C{-}C \leftarrow$ = single bond; $-C{=}C-$ = double bond; $-C{\equiv}C-$ = triple bond. Double and triple bonds are found in unsaturated compounds, single in saturated compounds.

Cartilage: gristle, a non-vascular elastic tissue, softer than bones.

Catabolism: see **metabolism**

Catalyst (catalysis): a substance (inorganic or organic) which increases the rate of a chemical reaction without undergoing any change itself.

Cataract: opacity of the crystalline lens of the eye, producing partial or total blindness.

Centrifugation: the process of separating solid material from solutions by rotating, at high speed, vessels containing the solution.

Cerebellar cortex: outer grey matter of the little or hind brain.

Cerebral cortex: outer grey matter of the brain.

Ceruloplasmin: copper-containing protein, a normal constituent of blood, said to protect the organism against copper poisoning.

Cheilosis: vertical lesions, complicated by redness, swelling and ulceration of the lips.

Cholesterol: a fat soluble steroid essential constituent of every animal cell and an essential nutrient factor, blood levels of cholesterol are often increased in coronary heart disease.

Chromatography: an analytical technique enabling separation of the components of a mixture by producing rates of movement for each component in a countercurrent system: movement of a liquid phase (solvent or eluent) over a stationary phase (adsorbent). See **column, thin layer** or **high pressure liquid chromatography**.

Circadian rhythm: daily cycle.

Co-enzyme % reactivation or effect: measures the stimulation that an *in vitro* addition of the vitamin co-enzyme has on the activity of the enzyme system in the erythrocytes; e.g. vitamin B_1 as TPP is the co-enzyme of transketolase (enzyme acting in carbohydrate metabolism); vitamin B_2 as FAD is the co-enzyme of glutathione reductase (enzyme acting in electron transfer); vitamin B_6 as PALP is the co-enzyme of glutamate oxaloacetate transaminase (enzyme acting in protein metabolism): The higher the % effect the more severe is the vitamin deficiency.

Co-enzymes or **co-factors** or **prosthetic groups** are non-protein organic compounds which in combination with the protein part of the enzyme (apoenzyme) play an intimate part in the catalysis by the enzyme (holo-enzyme).

Co-factors: see **co-enzymes**.

Colitis: inflammation of the colon which is part of the intestine.

Collagen: a constituent of connective tissue and the organic substance of bones: intercellular cement substance (it yields gelatin on boiling).

Column chromatography: the adsorbent is placed onto a column through which the solution of the mixture is fractionated using an appropriate solvent.

Conjunctiva: the mucous membrane connecting the inner eyelid and eyeball.

Conjunctivitis: inflammation of the conjunctiva.

Connective tissue of the body: fibrous tissue connecting and supporting the organs.

Corneal: of the cornea, the transparent horny part of the anterior covering of the eyeballs.

Coronary: two large arteries that branch from the aorta.

Corpus luteum: an ovarian follicle that has matured and discharged its ovum: it secretes progesterone.

Corticotropin (ACTH): adrenotropic hormone of the pituitary gland, maintains and controls the function of the adrenal cortex, affecting indirectly carbohydrate, protein and mineral metabolism.

Cortisone and hydrocortisone: steroid hormones produced by the adrenal cortex; enhance gluconeogenesis (catabolic process resulting in increased liver glycogen and blood sugar).

Coulter counter: an instrument enabling automatic blood cell count.

Creatine: a derivative of glycine. Cell constituent stored in muscles as phosphate.

Creatinine: the end product of creatine catabolism, normal constituent of urine.

Crohn's disease: regional enteritis and regional ileitis; inflammation of the terminal part of the ileum.

Crystallize: to separate from a solution into crystals.

Crystals (adjective **crystalline**): aggregation of molecules with a definite internal structure and external form of solids enclosed by symmetrically arranged plane faces.

Cyclic nucleotide: a nucleotide in which the phosphoric acid in the molecule is bridged onto the benzene ring.

Cystine: a naturally occurring amino acid, sometimes found in urine in form of hexagonal crystals; may form cystine calculi or stones.

Cytochrome c: enzyme in which the prosthetic group is an iron porphyrine, regarded as the universal catalyst of respiration, forming the essential electron-bridge between the respirable substrate and oxygen.

Cytochromes: electron transferring enzymes or oxidizing-reducing enzymes catalysing dehydrogenation or removal of electrons.

Deficiency (biochemical): absence or very low levels of a nutrient in the blood.

Deficiency state or clinical deficiency: a pathological condition resulting from a relative or absolute lack of an individual nutrient.

Dehydrogenases (aerobic and anaerobic): enzymes catalysing chiefly removal of hydrogen or of electrons from a molecule.

Detoxication: elimination of toxic substances by reaction.

Diabetes: see **insulin**.

Dicumarol: trade mark for a preparation of bis-hydroxy-coumarin, used as an anti-coagulant.

Dissociation constant (pK): see **ionization constant**.

Double blind trial: experiment in which both the patient(s) and the investigator(s) do not know which treatment the patient(s) are receiving, and a placebo preparation is used.

Double bond: see **carbon bonds**.

Ecchymosis: escape of blood into the tissues producing a blotchy area of discolouration.

Endocrine gland(s): glands that regulate the body functions by secretion of special hormones which are delivered into the blood.

Endogenous: formed or growing within e.g., the human body.

Enzyme (holo-enzyme): an organic catalyst formed by living cells, consisting of a protein (apo-enzyme) and a co-enzyme or co-factor or prosthetic group.

Epimer: an isomer differing from the other substance in the space orientation of the groups around the asymmetric carbon atom (usually occurring in sugars).

Epinephrine: see **adrenaline**.

Exogenous: formed or growing outside, e.g. the human body.

Extrapolate: in mathematics, to calculate from known terms of a series other terms which lie outside the range of the known terms.

Fluorimetry: method of analysis by which the fluorescence (luminescence) that a substance can emit, when excited, is measured.

Folic acid: one of the B-group vitamins (vitamin B_c), the deficiency of which causes macrocytic anaemia.

Follicles: pouch-like depressions or cavities.

Free radical: substance which contains an unpaired electron.

Functional tests: methods of analysis which determine a specific function of a metabolite (e.g. a vitamin which acts as co-enzyme: see **co-enzyme % reactivation or effect**).

Gamma rays: are the most penetrating of all types of rays; see **radiation**.

Gastric tube: rubber or plastic tube placed in the stomach to allow artificial feeding.

Gerocracy: meaning in the text the class of healthy old people.

Gingivitis: inflammation of the gums.

Glomerular: adjective of glomerulus.

Glomerular filtration: mechanism by which the kidneys eliminate water, products of catabolism and foreign substances.

Glomerulus (i): cluster of tissues or blood vessels, e.g. in kidneys.

Glutathione: a tripeptide containing glutamic acid, cystine and glycine, normal constituent of living cells: has coenzyme function in many enzymes: found in human blood but only in the erythrocytes.

Gum hypertrophy: enlarged swollen gums.

Haemodialysis (maintenance haemodialysis): an extrarenal procedure which allows blood purification by removing end-products of metabolism and replacing electrolytes such as sodium, potassium, carbon dioxide, calcium and other essential nutrients. Used in renal disease.

Haemoglobin: the oxygen-carrying pigment of the blood within the erythrocytes. It contains iron in the molecule.

Haemolysis: when the membranes of the erythrocytes break, haemoglobin (and other cell components) is released into the blood plasma, colouring it red. Assay of such plasma is invalid.

Half-life: the time interval during which the amount of a substance decreases by half.

Heavy metals: metals such as lead, mercury, arsenic, which are poisonous to man.

Hepatomegaly: enlarged liver detected by palpation of the abdomen.

Hess test: a small amount of the blue dye dicholophenolindophenol is placed on the skin and the time it takes to discolour indicates presence or absence of ascorbic acid.

High energy ionizing radiation: (e.g.) X-rays or gamma rays which by penetrating into a substance impart to it a certain amount of energy which it absorbs and through which changes in its atom(s) or molecule(s) occur, such as ionization.

High pressure liquid chromatography: quantitative chromatographic technique requiring minute quantities of sample. High pressure gas at room temperature is used to expel the eluent and hence the component(s) of the mixture to be fractionated out of the column with the adsorbent. The instrument is attached to a spectrophotometer allowing automatic and rapid measurement of the separated substances.

Histamine: see **anti-histamines**.

Homoeostatic (adjective of **Homoeostasis**): mechanism tending to keep biological system within a particular physiological range.

Hormones: substances formed in endocrine glands, serving to coordinate and stimulate some vital body processes.

Hydrocortisone: see **cortisone**.

Hydrolysis: a destructive process resulting in breakage of the molecule of a substance (e.g. polymers such as polysaccharides), caused by water, enzymes, bacteria etc.

Hydrophobic: averse to water, water-repellent.

Hydroxylation: transfer of OH group(s) from one molecule to another.

Hyperkeratosis: excessive thickening of the outer horny layer of the skin.

Hyperthyroidism: see **thyroidism**.

Incubation period: the interval of time required between the invasion of the body by a pathogenic organism and the appearance of the first symptoms of the disease.

Insulin: hormone produced by a group of cells called the islets of Langerhans situated in the pancreas. It acts as catalyst in the utilization of glucose by the various tissues either as a fuel for liberation of energy or as a store in the form of glycogen or fat. When the production of insulin is inadequate glucose accumulates rapidly in the blood and body fluids and when the concentration exceeds a certain point, glucose is excreted in the urine. This causes a waste of glucose and a pathological condition known as diabetes mellitus.

Interfacial tension: interface = boundary between two phases (e.g. liquid–liquid, solid–liquid); tension = the force existing at the interface between, e.g., two immiscible liquids such as oil and water.

Interferon: a protein produced by the interaction of animal cells and viruses that is capable of inhibiting virus multiplication.

Ions: electrically charged atoms which are transformed into positive ions (= cations) by the loss of an electron and into negative ions (= anions) by the gain of an electron.

Ionization: the dissociation of a molecule into electrically charged atoms, known as ions.

Ionization constant = dissociation constant = pK: the product of the concentration of the cation and of the anion divided by the concentration of the non-ionized molecule. This constant depends upon the solvent used and the temperature at which ionization occurs.

Irradiation: exposure to radiation or passage through an object or a substance of penetrating radiation.

Isomers: substances which have the same molecular formulae but differ from each other in the arrangement of the atoms (or radicals) in the molecule.

Isotopes: forms of the same element having identical atomic number but slightly different atomic weights; radioactive isotopes emit radiations which can be measured at some distance from the sample (e.g. carbon-14).

Jerks: involuntary spasmodic contraction of muscles.

Keratomalacia: characteristic softening of the entire thickness of part or mostly whole of the cornea leading to perforation and iris prolapse (slipping out of place of the coloured membrane of the eye).

Ketosugar: a sugar containing a keto group = CO.

Koilonychia: bilateral, spoon-shaped deformity of nails, occurring in older children and adults.

Korsakoff's syndrome or psychosis: a confusion state with confabulation and polyneuritis thought to be due to vitamin B_1 deficiency.

Kyphoscoliosis: hunch formation accompanied by lateral curvature of the spine.

Labelled: e.g. ^{14}C-labelled ascorbic acid (AA): the isotope of carbon of atomic weight 14 is introduced in the AA molecule to serve as tracer, e.g. for studying

AA absorption and metabolism. This AA is administered orally or by injection and the radioactivity it emits can be easily measured.

Labial: of the lips.

Labile: unstable, liable to change.

Laryngitis: inflammation of the larynx = the voice box = muscular and cartilagenous structure lined with mucous membranes, situated at the top of the windpipe and below the root of the tongue.

Lesion: damage, injury, morbid change in the texture or function of tissues or organs.

ad Libitum: at choice and as much as wanted.

Lipoid: fat.

Load test: administration of a large dose of a substance, under standard conditions, to determine absorption, metabolism and excretion.

Lumen in physiology: space, cavity.

Malabsorption: insufficient absorption of nutritive substances by the intestinal mucosa, due to various causes.

Malaise: bodily discomfort, without development of a specific disease.

Malaria (swampfever, cold fever): intermittent and remittent fever caused by bite of the anopheles mosquito which conveys the infectious germ (plasmodium). The germ penetrates into the blood erythrocytes where it grows and multiplies.

Marsupials: animals with a pouch in which to carry their young, born imperfect.

Matrix: formative part of an animal tissue or organ (e.g. bones).

Megaloblastic anaemia: anaemic condition detected by presence of abnormal erythrocytes, large and with a nucleus.

Melanin: complex pigment found in dark skin and dark human hair.

Melting point: a pure crystalline substance melts at a constant temperature, at a given pressure; it may decompose in the process.

Membrane permeability: ability of the membrane to let substances diffuse through itself.

Metabolism: the process in an organism or a single cell by which nutritive material is built up into living matter = constructive metabolism = **anabolism** or alternatively the process by which the material is broken down into simpler substances to perform special functions = destructive metabolism = **catabolism**.

Metabolite: a substance which takes part in metabolic pathways.

Methylcellulose: a methyl ($-CH_3$) ester of cellulose used as a bulking agent and a suspending agent.

Methylglyoxal: CH_3COCHO, a dark green liquid which undergoes polymerization very easily (i.e. it reacts with itself to form larger molecules). It is easily converted to lactic acid by several enzymes.

Microcytic anaemia: anaemic condition detected by the presence of abnormally small erythrocytes.

Moiety: a part or portion: e.g. reducing moiety or oxidizing moiety.

Myocardium: the muscular substance of the heart.

Myotatic: muscle sensitive to touch.

Neoplastic cells: cancer cells.

Nicotinamide adenine dinucleotide (NAD): co-enzyme of many dehydrogenases in which function the pyridine ring of the molecule is reduced to NADH.

Night blindness: the inability to see well at night (to adapt to darkness), due to vitamin A deficiency.

Nitrosamines: toxic substances formed by the action of nitrites (e.g. in food) on a variety of amines at the pH range of the mammalian stomach.

Noradrenaline (norepinephrine): demethylated precursor of adrenaline (epinephrine).

Nucleic acids: polynucleotides; RNA, the cell messenger, is found in the cell fluid (cytoplasm) and some in the cell nucleus; DNA is found in the nucleus of the cell: on the sequence of nucleotides in its molecule appears to lie the chemical basis for heredity.

Nucleoside: formed by a sugar and a heterocyclic (having e.g. some N instead of C atoms in the rings) base (e.g. purine, pyrimidine derivatives).

Nucleotide: a nucleoside esterified with phosphoric acid: nucleosides occur in all living cells and are precursor of nucleic acids.

Nystagmus: continual movement of the eyeballs.

Ocular: of the eye.

Oestrogens: female hormones which stimulate or regulate growth and development of the uterus and other membranes.

Optical isomer: isomers which differ from each other in their ability (**optical activity**) to rotate the plane of polarized light (= light exhibiting different properties in different directions at right angles to the line of propagation).

Optical rotation: a physical property of certain substances which possess structural asymmetry to rotate the plane of polarized light.

Oral: of the mouth.

Oral lichen planus: a common skin condition which exhibits lesions in the mouth.

Oxidases: enzymes that catalyse oxidation reactions.

Oxidation: an increase in positive charges on an atom or the loss of negative charges (opposite to reduction).

Palsies (of nerves): paralyses.

Pancreas: large gland located below and behind the stomach and liver; it secretes **insulin**.

Papillae (adjective papillary): small nipple-like elevations in the tongue.

Parameters: in biochemistry and haematology: constant components of blood plasma, serum or blood cells: e.g. urea, total protein, haemoglobin, blood cell count.

Paraplegia: paralysis of lower limbs and part or whole of the trunk.

Parkinson's disease: paralysis agitans.

Pedometer: instrument for estimating distance travelled on foot and recording numbers of steps taken.

Pellagra: deficiency disease due to lack of vitamin PP (nicotinic acid. nicotinamide), characterized by cracking of skin, diarrhoea and insanity. Can cause death.

Perifollicular: around the follicles.

Peripheral neuropathy: pathological condition of the peripheral nerves (i.e. the portion of the nervous system outside the brain and the spinal cord).

Peritoneal cavity: the space between the two layers lining the walls of the abdominal and pelvic cavities.

Peroxidases: oxidizing enzymes which catalyse reactions leading to release of energy.

Petechiae: small round haemorrhagic spots in skin and mucous membranes.

pH range: pH expresses the degree to which a solution is acidic or alkaline and extends from 0 for 'pure' acid to 14 for 'pure' base. pH = 7 indicates neutrality (water); a pH of less than 7 indicates acidity, and of more than 7 alkalinity.

Phagocytosis: a body defence mechanism by which e.g. the leukocytes go to the site of infection, circulate and ingest the infectious micro-organism and destroy it within their cells.

Phosphodiesterase: enzyme which hydrolyses mono- and di-phosphoric esters and has the ability of breaking the lactone ring of a molecule.

Phospholipids: fatty acid derivatives containing phosphate.

Photosynthesis: formation (creation) of new substances activated by sunlight.

Pituitary: called the master gland of the endocrine system because it controls the hormone production of other endocrine glands.

Placebo: a preparation (e.g. tablet, capsule) identical in appearance and taste to that containing a therapeutic agent but without it; used in double blind clinical trials for negative control purposes to test efficacy of the therapeutic agent, independently from psychological factors accompanying the administration.

Planar: on a surface; two-dimensional.

Plasma threshold value (renal plasma clearance) (C): relationship between concentration of a substance in the urine (*U*) and plasma (*P*) in mg/l and the rate (*V*) of urinary excretion in ml/minute: $C = (U \times V)/P$.

Platelets: or thrombocytes: small disc- or plate-like cells, the smallest of the formed elements of blood; involved in blood coagulation.

Pneumonia: acute inflammation or infection of the lungs.

Porphyria: metabolic abnormality in which porphyrin (the iron-free derivative of haemoglobin) appears in the urine.

Proliferation: cells reproduce themselves and grow by multiplication of elementary parts.

Prophylactic: adjective of **prophylaxis**: tending to ward off disease.

Prosthetic group: see **co-enzyme**.

Prothrombin time: the time taken by blood to coagulate; it reveals changes in coagulation factors of the plasma and is used to check the action of oral anticoagulants.

Psychomotor: inducing movement by mental action.

Purine: see **uric acid**.

Pyorrhoea: profound changes in the gums.

Radiation: emission of electromagnetic rays (heat rays, rays of light) by certain power sources such as hot globar element (IR-rays); Na lamp (visible light); H or Hg lamp (UV rays); electrons (X-rays); radio-isotopes (gamma rays). All these rays are electromagnetic and differ from each other in the frequency and wavelength.

Redox potential: electrical constant, characteristic of those substances which act in reduced and oxidized form, in giving away or receiving electrons or hydrogen atoms. It is measured by reference to the H–H ion couple (electrode) as zero and depends upon concentration of electrons or atoms and temperature.

Reduction: an increase in the negative charges of an atom or a loss of positive charges (opposite to oxidation).

'Reference' adult man: the ideal man over 18 years of age weighing 70 kg and of 172 cm height.

'Reference' adult woman: the ideal woman over 18 years of age weighing 50 kg and of 162 cm height.

Renal: pertaining to the kidneys.

Renal plasma clearance: see **plasma threshold value**.

Re-saturation: replenish with a nutrient an organism which was deprived of it.

Retina: layer at the back of the eyeball, sensitive to light.

Rhagades: painful fissuring of lips and skin.

Rheumatoid arthritis: chronic inflammatory disease of the joints.

Rhinitis: inflammation of the mucous membrane of the nose.

Rhinovirus: virus affecting the mucous membrane of the nose.

Saturation in chemistry: the state of a solvent that holds in solution all of a substance it can possibly contain; in physiology **tissue saturation** means that the tissues retain the greatest amount possible of a substance.

Schizophrenia: mental disease marked by disconnection between thoughts, feelings and actions.

Seborrhoea: abnormal scaling of the skin.

Single blind trial (see **double blind trial**): in this case only the patient(s) does not know the treatment; alternatively no placebo preparation is used as control.

Sinus: eight cavities in the skull that are connected with the nasal cavity.

Skinfold: double layer of skin and subcutaneous fat: it is measured by means of a caliper.

Slurry free flowing: semiliquid or semisolid homogenized mixture which can be poured easily.

Spinal cord: cylindrical structure within the canal of the spine; part of the nervous system.

Spinal fluid: liquid constituent which surrounds and protects the spinal cord.

Spleen: large gland-like organ situated under the ribs in the upper left quadrant of the abdomen.

Standard oxidation–reduction potential: see **redox potential**.

Steady state: condition at which plasma and tissue concentrations of vitamin C remain at a constant level.

Steroids: complex, fat soluble molecules of characteristic structure, among which are cholesterol, vitamins D_2 and D_3, sex hormones; they contain only C, H and O.

Sub-scapular: under the shoulder blade.

Supernatant: the liquid remaining on top of the solid sediment after centrifugation of a suspension.

Sustained release preparations (e.g. capsules): products contained in capsules, intended to provide prolonged therapeutic action after oral administration.

Synergism: active participation in a reaction of two or more substances having the same properties (opposite to antagonism).

Therapy: curative treatment.

Thermodynamic equilibrium in physics: state of balance between mechanical work and heat; in physiology: refers to reactions occurring under normal conditions.

Thin layer chromatography: a simple quantitative chromatographic method in which a drop of the sample solution is applied onto a thin layer of adsorbent which is spread evenly over a glass plate. This is placed vertically in a chamber with the appropriate eluent which, in ascending manner, will develop the chromatogram.

Thrombin: an enzyme resulting from the activation of prothrombin which catalyses the conversion of fibrinogen to fibrin. Fibrinogen is a high weight protein in the blood plasma which takes part in blood clotting.

Thrombosis: blocking of blood vessels by a blood clot.

Thymus: a two lobed ductless gland situated behind the upper part of the sternum and extending into the neck. It is a fairly large gland in childhood and usually shrinks in adulthood.

Thyroid: shield-shaped large ductless gland which secretes the hormone thyroxin.

Thyroidism: hyperthyroidism: excessive functioning of the thyroid gland; **hypothyroidism:** reduced functioning of the thyroid gland = goitre = thyroid enlargement.

Thyroxin: contains iodine in the molecule and is essential for normal metabolism and development see **thyroid**.

Tissue saturation: see **saturation**.

Tonsillitis: inflammation of the tonsils (two organs on each side of the fauces, cavity at the back of the mouth).

Toxic: poisonous, pertaining to poison.

Transaminases: enzymes which catalyse the transfer of amino groups from one molecule to another.

Transferrin: a protein present in blood serum and liver which is active in the transport of iron in ferric(III) form.

Trauma: morbid condition of the body produced by wound, violence or emotional shock.

Triceps: large three-headed muscle of the back of the arm.

Tubular: pertaining to kidney tubes.

Turnover in physiology: amount of a substance (e.g. ascorbic acid) which is turned over in the body per day. (Under steady state conditions it is equal to the amount of ascorbic acid which is absorbed per day.)

Ubiquitous: universally or widely distributed.

Ultraviolet (UV) absorption, UV spectrum: see **absorption spectrum**.

Urea: a product of protein metabolism.

Uric acid: the end product of purine metabolism. Purine is an organic heterocyclic base containing 4 atoms of nitrogen instead of carbon in the rings; basic component of nucleosides and nucleotides.

Vascular: pertaining to blood vessels.

Virus: a minute infectious agent that requires susceptible host cells for multiplication.

Vitamins: micro-nutrients; organic compounds which are required for normal growth and maintenance of life of animals and man and cannot, as a rule, be synthesized within the body, but must be obtained from food. They do not furnish energy but are essential for the transformation of energy within the body, i.e. for the metabolism of carbohydrate, fat and protein, and for the regulation of metabolic processes. Fat-soluble vitamins are: **Vitamin A** (alcohol, aldehyde and esters also called retinol, retinaldehyde, retinyl esters) – the provitamin A **beta carotene** is converted in the body to vitamin A; **Vitamins D_2** (calciferol, ergocalciferol) and **D_3** (cholecalciferol); **Vitamin E** (tocopherols); **Vitamins K_1** and **K_2**. Water-soluble vitamins are: **Vitamin B_1** (thiamine); **Vitamin B_2** (riboflavin); **Vitamin PP** (nicotinic acid and nicotinamide); **Vitamin B_3** or **B_5** (pantothenic acid); **Vitamin B_6** (pyridoxine, pyridoxal, pyridoxamine); **Vitamin B_{12}** (cyanocobalamin); **Vitamin H** (biotin); **Vitamin B_c** (folic acid); **Vitamin C** (L-ascorbic acid, monodehydro-L-ascorbic acid and dehydro-L-ascorbic acid).

in Vitro: (experiment or reaction) done in the laboratory.

in Vivo: (reaction) occurring within the body.

Warfarin: a compound used as an anti-coagulant in the form of sodium or potassium salts.

Wernicke's encephalopathy: (encephalic = of the brain) acute vitamin B_1 deficiency resulting in mental confusion and nystagmus.

Xerophthalmia: inflammation of the conjunctiva of the eye with abnormal dryness and thickening of the skin, which can lead to blindness and is due to deficiency of vitamin A.

Xerosis: generalized dryness of the skin with branny scaling.

X-rays: see **radiation**.

Index

AA *see* ascorbic acid
abbreviations 161, 162
aboriginals
  malnutrition 80
  plasma vitamin C levels 80, 81
absorption 57–9
acidosis and megadoses 128
ackee, vitamin C assessment 44
adrenal glands 12, 14
  vitamin C content 61
adrenaline synthesis 12, 66
age
  and vitamin C content of tissue 59, 61
  vitamin C intake and plasma levels 101, 103
alcohol and vitamin C status 106, 135
alcoholism 84, 86, 135
  blood vitamin C profiles 86
  and recommended dose 110
alkali and optical rotation 21
allergies 135
amino acid
  hydrolysis 12
  metabolism 66
AMP, cyclic
  levels and vitamin C levels 123
  protection 26, 66, 121
AMP phosphodiesterase 121
anaemia 84, 135
  megaloblastic 79, 127
animals and ability to synthesize vitamin C 17, 18
antioxidant properties 38
antiscorbutic factor
  isolation 16
  and origin of name 18
apples
  cooking 40, 41
  dried 41
  eating 40
  vitamin C assessment 40, 41, 54
apricots, vitamin C assessment 41
artichokes, vitamin C assessment 44
L-2-ascorbate sulphate 62
  in urine 64
L-ascorbic acid (AA) 10, 21
  absorption properties 21
  and cancer 124, 125
  and common cold 113–15, 118–23, 126
    duration 124
    onset 124
    trial variables 122, 123
  diuretic 128
  ionization in water 23
  main component in body 25, 64
  megadoses 125–31
  metal complexing 25
  oxidation 23
  oxidation products 24
  physico-chemical properties 21, 22
  positive optical rotation 21
  redox potential 22, 23
  stability in plasma 25
  stability in water 23
  structural formula 12, 13
  therapeutic uses 111–31
ascorbic acid in biochemical assay interference 130
ascorbic acid oxidase 26
asparagus, vitamin C assessment 44
aspirin, effect on vitamin C levels 107, 122
assay methods
  biological 28
  blood 29
  chromatographic 29, 30
  dichlorphenolindophenol 28
  fluorimetry 29, 30, 137, 138
  food 27–9
  human tissue 29, 30

physicochemical 28
plasma 29
precautions 27
sample preparation 27–30, 137
urine 29
assessment of status 97–104
biochemical 99–101
clinical 97, 98, 100, 101
dietary 98–101
atherosclerosis, vitamin C and 125, 135
avocado pears, vitamin C assessment 41
aubergine, vitamin C assessment 44

bananas, vitamin C assessment 41
beans, vitamin C assessment 44, 45
bean sprouts, vitamin C assessment 45
beetroot, vitamin C assessment 45
beri-beri 15
vitamin C levels 83, 84
vitamin profile 84
beverages, vitamin C assessment 39, 54
bilberries, vitamin C assessment 41
biochemical function 18
biochemical reactivity 24–6
biological activities 12
biosynthesis
ability of animals 17, 18
and evolution 19
birds, location of vitamin C enzyme system 17, 18
blackberries, vitamin C assessment 41
blackcurrant juice 37
vitamin C assessment 40
blackcurrants, vitamin C assessment 41
blanching, effects on vitamin C 33, 34
blood
dietary and biochemical vitamin C status 102
vitamin C content 62
body fluids
vitamin C assay 29, 30
see also blood, plasma, urine
body pool, vitamin C 60
bottling, effects on vitamin C 34
brains
vitamin C assessment 49
vitamin C content and age 59
bread improvement 38
broccoli, vitamin C assessment 45
brussels sprouts, vitamin C assessment 45
buffy coat 30
vitamin C content 59, 60, 62

cabbage
shredding and vitamin C loss 32
vitamin C assessment 45
calcium metabolism 67
calories
foodstuffs 39, 51
Italian menu 142, 143
typical British menu 142, 143
vegetarian menu 141
cancer and vitamin C status 124, 125, 135
canning, effects on vitamin C 34
carrots, vitamin C assessment 46
catarrh 120
cauliflower, vitamin C assessment 46
celeriac, vitamin C assessment 46
celery, vitamin C assessment 46
cevitamic acid 16
chemical formulae 16
cherries, vitamin C assessment 41
chicory, vitamin C assessment 46
chromatography
high-pressure liquid 29, 30
thin layer 38
circadian rhythm and vitamin C metabolism 57, 58
climate
cold and recommended dose 92, 108
and vitamin C requirements 107, 108, 135
clinical assessment 97, 98
coenzyme role 14
collagen formation 12, 66
common cold (acute rhinitis)
ascorbic acid and 113–15, 118, 121, 126
assessment of vitamin C role 121–4
causes 112, 113
clinical trials 114–16
leukocyte depletion of vitamin C 117, 118
low temperature exposure 120
and malfunctioning 120
molecular biology 119–24
prevention 115
sex differences 117
symptoms 113, 117, 122

vitamin C, biochemical effects 115–19
and vitamin C metabolism 117
conjunctiva lesions and scurvy diagnosis 71
cooking, effects of institutional and home on vitamin C 36
copper metabolism 12, 25, 66
courgette (zucchini), vitamin C assessment 46, 49
cranberries, vitamin C assessment 41
Crohn's disease 73
cucumber, vitamin C assessment 46
currants, vitamin C assessment of dried 41; *see also* black and redcurrants
cytochrome C reduction 66

daily intake 87–96
in common cold 119
needed 60, 63
recommendations 109, 110
supplemented 77
variable recommendations 87
dates, vitamin C assessment 41
dehydro-L-ascorbic acid (DHAA) 10, 21
antiscorbutic activity 18
and cell division 25
fat solubility 25
formation 17
hydrophobic 25
occurrence in body 65
oxidation and hydration 13
positive optical rotation 21
redox potential 24
reduction 23
structural formula 12, 13
deficiency
clinical 100
dangers 70
developmental stages 74
effects of 68–73
and health 83
and plasma levels 91
vitamin B_1 85
see also hypovitaminosis, scurvy
detoxication 67
DHAA *see* dehydro-L-ascorbic acid
diabetes, vitamin C levels 25, 135
2,6-dichlorphenol indophenol 28
diet
Italian, vitamin C content 142, 143
typical British, vitamin C content 139, 140
vegetarian, vitamin C and calories 141
dietary allowances
based on scurvy prevention 90–3
FAO/WHO 91–3
infants and children, US 95
international comparisons 92, 94, 96
pregnancy and lactation 90, 94
and tissue saturation 93, 94
UK 90, 91
variability 94–6
vitamin C, US 89
dietary assessment 98, 99
2,4-dinitrophenylhydrazine 29
diketo-L-gulonic acid 24
discovery of vitamin C 15–20
disease
vitamin C effects in 113–25
vitamin C functions in 119
and vitamin C levels 82–4, 135
distribution, vitamin C in man 58–63
dose and good health 10
double bonds and absorption spectra 21–3
drugs
and vitamin C status 135
and vitamin C tissue desaturation 106, 107

elderly, vitamin C repletion, effects 78, 79
endive, vitamin C assessment 46
enrichment 37, 38
erythorbic acid, antioxidant 38
erythrocytes
coenzyme reactivation 84–6
vitamin C content 62
evolutionary process and vitamin C biosynthesis 19
excretion
urinary 63
vitamin C in man 58, 63, 64

FAO/WHO recommended daily doses 91–3
figs, vitamin C assessment 41
fluorimetric determination 29, 30, 137, 138

folic acid, dietary allowance 81
folic acid metabolism 12, 66
food
  animal 35, 36
  empty calorie 56
  as source 11
  storage and cooking methods 31
  vegetable 31–5
  vitamin C in 31–56
  vitamin C assay tables 27–9, 38–55
  vitamin C points 53
  see also individual foodstuffs
Food Composition Tables, symbols 52, 53
fortification 37, 38
freeze-drying 35
freezing and vitamin C preservation 35
fruit 15
fruit juices, vitamin C content 36, 37
function of vitamin C 64–75
future research 133–6

glutathione 25, 67
GMP, cyclic, protection 26, 66
gooseberries, vitamin C assessment 42
grapefruit, vitamin C assessment 42
grapefruit juice 37
  vitamin C assessment 39
grapes, vitamin C assessment 42
guavas, vitamin C assessment 42
guinea pigs
  vitamin C deficient and assay 28
L-gulono-γ-lactone oxidase
  location in animals 17
  loss in humans 17

half-life 62
  and dose 63
health and vitamin C levels 83
heart, vitamin C assessment 49
hexuronic acid 16
horseradish, vitamin C assessment 46
humans, inability to synthesise vitamin C 17, 18
hydrogen ions, donation and receipt 18, 19
hyperkeratosis 71, 72
hyperthyroidism and vitamin C levels 25
hypovitaminosis C
  Australian case studies 77–86
  plasma levels 81, 83, 84
  prevention and cure 73–5
  socioeconomic stress groups 81, 82

infertility 129
insulin 26
intake and plasma levels
  effect of age and sex 101, 103
interactions 67
Iowa studies 70–3
  and FAO/WHO recommendations 91
iron metabolism 12, 25, 66
isolation 16

jam and marmalade, vitamin C content 34, 51

kidney
  reabsorption 63, 64
  site of synthesis 17, 19
  vitamin C assessment 50

labile pool 57
lactation, recommended dose 90, 94
lactone ring 21, 22
leeks, vitamin C assessment 46
lemon juice 37
lemons, vitamin C assessment 42
lentils, vitamin C assessment 46
lettuce, vitamin C assessment 46
leukocytes 30
  excess vitamin C storage 101, 102
  vitamin C content 62
lichen planus 86
limes, vitamin C assessment 42
liver
  site of vitamin C synthesis 17, 19
  vitamin C assessment 50, 60
loganberries, vitamin C assessment 42
lychees, vitamin C assessment 42
L-lyxonic acid 24

magnesium metabolism 25
malnutrition 82
  vitamin 84
  and vitamin C levels 83
mandarins, vitamin C assessment 42
mangoes, vitamin C assessment 42, 43
marrow, vitamin C assessment 47
MDHAA *see* monodehydro-L-ascorbic acid

meals-on-wheels
  orange juice supplement 79
  and vitamin C 79
meat, vitamin C assessment 54
mechanism of action 14
megadoses 125–31
  and acidosis 127
  biochemical assay interference 130
  drug interactions 129
  gastrointestinal effects 126
  nutrient interactions 127
  oxaluria 128
  and stones 128, 129
  withdrawal syndrome 129, 130
melons, vitamin C assessment 43
melting points, vitamin C system 22, 23
  mental performance
  and meals-on-wheels in elderly 78, 79
  and vitamin C levels in elderly 77, 78
  and vitamin C repletion 78
metabolism, vitamin C
  body pool contribution 57
  during common cold 117
  proportion of intake 91
  relationships of 133, 134
metabolites, excretion of 64
metaphosphoric acid and sample preparation 27–9
methylglyoxal 14
milk
  human and infant tissue saturation 89
  vitamin C assessment 50, 51, 54
  vitamin C in breast 35, 36
monodehydro-L-ascorbic acid (MDHAA) 10, 21
  absorption properties 21
  antiscorbutic activity 18
  biochemical reactivity 26
  in catarrah 120
  chemical formula 16
  free radical 17, 24, 26
  intermediate role 16
  physicochemical properties 21, 22
  redox potential 22, 24
  structural formula 13
mulberries, vitamin C assessment 43
mushrooms, vitamin C assessment 47
mustard and cress, vitamin C assessment 47

NADH-dependent oxidase 66
nectarines, vitamin C assessment 43
nitrosamine detoxication 67
nomenclature 18, 20
nutritional interrelationships 133

okra, vitamin C assessment 47
olives, vitamin C assessment 43
onions, vitamin C assessment 47
optical rotation 21, 22
oral contraceptives 107, 122
  and recommended daily dose 110
orange juice 37
  vitamin C assessment 39, 40
oranges, vitamin C assessment 43
oxaluria 128

parsley, vitamin C assessment 47
parsnips, vitamin C assessment 47
passion fruit, vitamin C assessment 43
paw paw, vitamin C assessment 43
peach, vitamin C assessment 43
pears, vitamin C assessment 43
peas, vitamin C content and processing 33, 47
peppers, vitamin C assessment 47
petechiae 71
pH
  cooking media 34
  and oxidation products 24
pineapple, vitamin C assessment 43
pineapple juice 37
  vitamin C assessment 40
plantain, vitamin C assessment 47
plasma
  levels as index 88, 91
  threshold value 63
  vitamin C content 62
    and sex 60
  vitamin C determination 137, 138
  vitamin C levels, classification 101
platelets, vitamin C content 62
plums, vitamin C assessment 43
pollution 135
pomegranates, vitamin C assessment 43
potato crisps, vitamin C assessment 48
potatoes and vitamin C
  assessment 47, 48, 54
  fortification 37
  loss and cooking method 33, 48
  loss during storage 32, 33, 48

potato powder, vitamin C assessment 48
pregnancy, recommended doses 90, 94
preservation 24
preservatives and vitamin C loss 35
proline hydroxylation 66
properties of vitamin C 11
protein, waking of dormant 14
prunes, vitamin C assessment 43
pumpkin, vitamin C assessment 48
Pure Food Act, New South Wales (1977) 36

quince, vitamin C assessment 44

radish, vitamin C assessment 48
raisins, vitamin C assessment 44
raspberries, vitamin C assessment 44
red currants, vitamin C assessment 41
redox potentials, vitamin C system 22–4
redox system, vitamin C 22
composition 10, 21
function 64–75
instability 27
plants and animals 11, 12
structural formulae 11–13
relationships, biochemical of vitamin C 14
renal calculi 128, 129
oxalate 128
research, future 133–6
restoration of vitamin C losses 37
rheumatoid arthritis 107
rhubarb, vitamin C assessment 44
roe, vitamin C assessment 50, 54
rosehip syrup, vitamin C assessment 40

saliva, vitamin C content 62
salsify, vitamin C assessment 48
scalding, effects on vitamin C 33, 34
scorbutico 75
scurvy 15, 16
aboriginal babies 80
Australian case study 77–86
blood vitamin profile 86
clinical diagnosis 69
infantile 73, 129
Iowa study 70–3
mental changes 72, 73
minimum protective dose of vitamin C 69, 70
ocular lesions, timing 68
prevention and cure 68–75, 111
prevention in elderly 79
prevention and tissue saturation 88–90
preventatives 15
Sheffield study 69, 70
signs and symptoms 71
variation in symptom development 72
and vitamin C deficiency 74
vitamin C needed to replenish 60, 70
vitamin C pool in 60
see also hypovitaminosis, deficiency
seakale, vitamin C assessment 48
serum, vitamin C content 62
sex, vitamin C intake and plasma levels 101, 103
Sheffield study 69, 70
side effects of megadoses 124, 126–30
silverbeet, vitamin C assessment 48
smoking
and recommended dose 110
and vitamin C levels 105, 106, 122, 136
socioeconomic stress groups 81–3
sodium ascorbate, physicochemical properties 21, 22
solubility 11, 31, 32
sources of vitamin C 11, 38–54
spinach, vitamin C assessment 48
spring greens, vitamin C assessment 48
stability 12, 22, 23
and preservation 24
stable pool 57
steroids, synthesis of anti-inflammatory 66
storage
and intake 89
vitamin C in man 58
strawberries, vitamin C assessment 44
structure of vitamin C 21
Stucky points 53
sultanas, vitamin C assessment 44
sweat and excretion 62, 63
swedes, vitamin C assessment 49
sweetbread, vitamin C assessment 50
sweet corn, vitamin C assessment 49
sweet potatoes, vitamin C assessment 49
symbols 162

synthesis
  industrial 16
  and origin of life 14

tangerines, vitamin C assessment 44
therapeutic effects of vitamin C 111–31
L-threonic acid 24
L-threo-2,3,4,5,6 pentahydroxy-1-hexenoic acid-4-lactone 16
tissue
  damage and vitamin C loss 32, 34
  levels in stress 123
  saturation 88–90, 93, 94
    in common cold 118
  vitamin C assay 29, 30
  vitamin C content 35, 36
  vitamin C saturation values 62
  vitamin C storage 59, 62, 120
tissue synthesis, and plasma levels of vitamin C 89
tomatoes, vitamin C assessment 49
tomato juice, vitamin C assessment 40
tomato puree, vitamin C assessment 51, 54
tomato sauce, vitamin C assessment 51
tongue, vitamin C assessment 50
tripe, vitamin C assessment 50
turnips, vitamin C assessment 49

ultraviolet, effects on vitamin C system 23
ultraviolet absorption spectra 21, 22
urine
  vitamin C assessment 39
  vitamin C content 62, 100

vegetables
  shoot tips 54
  vitamin C content 44–9
vitamin, origin of word 15
vitamin A
  pro-, deficiency 86, 106
  sugar enrichment 37
vitamin B
  deficiencies 85, 86, 106
  metabolism 66
vitamin C, use of word 18, 20
vitamin E synergism 66
vitamin metabolism and vitamin C interaction 12

watercress, vitamin C assessment 49
Wernicke's encephalopathy, blood vitamin profile 85
withdrawal syndrome 129, 130
worm infestation 81
wound healing 12, 89

xerophthalmia 15
X-rays 23
L-xylonic acid 24

GPSR Compliance

The European Union's (EU) General Product Safety Regulation (GPSR) is a set of rules that requires consumer products to be safe and our obligations to ensure this.

If you have any concerns about our products, you can contact us on ProductSafety@springernature.com

In case Publisher is established outside the EU, the EU authorized representative is:

Springer Nature Customer Service Center GmbH
Europaplatz 3
69115 Heidelberg, Germany

Batch number: 10830943

Printed by Printforce, the Netherlands